SpringerBriefs in Public Health

SpringerBriefs in Public Health present concise summaries of cutting-edge research and practical applications from across the entire field of public health, with contributions from medicine, bioethics, health economics, public policy, biostatistics, and sociology.

The focus of the series is to highlight current topics in public health of interest to a global audience, including health care policy; social determinants of health; health issues in developing countries; new research methods; chronic and infectious disease epidemics; and innovative health interventions.

Featuring compact volumes of 55 to 125 pages, the series covers a range of content from professional to academic. Possible volumes in the series may consist of timely reports of state-of-the art analytical techniques, reports from the field, snapshots of hot and/or emerging topics, literature reviews, and in-depth case studies. Both solicited and unsolicited manuscripts are considered for publication in this series.

Briefs are published as part of Springer's eBook collection, with millions of users worldwide. In addition, Briefs are available for individual print and electronic purchase.

Briefs are characterized by fast, global electronic dissemination, standard publishing contracts, easy-to-use manuscript preparation and formatting guidelines, and expedited production schedules. We aim for publication 8–12 weeks after acceptance.

Valerie Chang Greer • Linda S. Edelman
Editors

Age-Friendly Ecosystems

Environments for Equitable Aging by Design

Springer

Editors
Valerie Chang Greer
College of Architecture and Planning,
School of Architecture,
Healthy Aging and Resilient Places Lab
The University of Utah
Salt Lake City, UT, USA

Linda S. Edelman
College of Nursing, Hartford Center of
Geriatric Nursing Excellence,
Utah Geriatric Education Consortium
(UGEC), Utah Rural Opioid Consortium
Collaborative Care Model (UROHC-CCM)
The University of Utah
Salt Lake City, UT, USA

ISSN 2192-3698 ISSN 2192-3701 (electronic)
SpringerBriefs in Public Health
ISBN 978-3-031-68360-2 ISBN 978-3-031-68361-9 (eBook)
https://doi.org/10.1007/978-3-031-68361-9

This Springer imprint is published by the registered company Springer Nature Switzerland AG
The registered company address is: Gewerbestrasse 11, 6330 Cham, Switzerland

For our elders—our parents, grandparents, aunts and uncles who model aging well—and for the next generation who follow in this journey; and for Isla.

Foreword

Whether referred to as age-friendly city (WHO 2007), livable community (e.g., Oberlink 2008), or age-friendly community (Lui et al. 2009), the early part of this twenty-first century has been characterized by growing advocacy for making "environments and systems within localities more supportive of long and healthy lives" (Greenfield and Buffel 2022: 1). Diaz Moore, Scharlach and Greenfield (2018) recognize that age-friendly community initiatives (AFCIs) get defined differently, but generally are collaborative, interdisciplinary or interprofessional efforts to change the physical setting—such as initiatives like visitability (Pynoos et al. 2010) and complete streets (LaPlante and McCann 2008)—or policy to enhance independence or mobility of older individuals (Golant 2015), or to provide supportive programs within naturally occurring retirement communities, such as the Villages concept (Village to Village 2015). They go on to advocate for a place-based approach to understanding and creating age-friendly communities, with place understood as a core concept from environmental gerontology that integrates people, program and the physical setting (Diaz Moore 2014).

Terry Fulmer, president of the John A. Hartford Foundation, suggests a reframing of age-friendly communities as "eco-systems" (this volume), which here has been conceptualized as involving rethinking of neighborhoods, campuses and health systems. The twentieth-century manifestation of these places was informed by shared paradigmatic assumptions such as: subsequent generational growth, unlimited natural resources, functional differentiation and medicine being more focused on cure than care (Diaz Moore in press). Yet we now find ourselves at a tipping point with age-related communities not proving sustainable, subsequent generations now shrinking, and a climate crisis unrelentingly drawer closer.

Aging in the Twenty-First Century Intermountain West

Nowhere is this more evident than in Utah and the Intermountain West, where we see climate impacts on our air quality and water scarcity and our approach to urbanization typified by twentieth-century suburbanization strategies that now strain the resilience of our ecology. Given this confluence, it should not be surprising that Phoenix, one of the fastest growing metropolises in America, recently announced a development moratorium (Healy 2023). Similar conversations have begun in Utah as well, highlighted by a dropping water level in the Great Salt Lake exposing toxic arsenic-laced dust that becomes airborne and threatens the populous Salt Lake Valley (Osborne 2023). A warming planet is also increasing air pollution arising from wildfires, another negative impact on cardiopulmonary health. Additionally, the confluence of our mountainous terrain and prevailing weather patterns creates moments of inversion where GHG emissions are trapped in the valley atmosphere and are associated with lost school/workdays and increased hospital admissions (Errigo et al. 2020).

The drop in Great Salt Lake levels is indicative of over-usage of water occurring during the current drought in the region. While some conservation methods have been enacted, the region's projected growth will place 7 of 11 water basins into high or very high stress criticality levels (Khatri et al. 2018). Interestingly, climate models suggest an overall increase in precipitation, but that precipitation is likely to come in fewer but more substantial rain/snow events, likely leading to reduced effectiveness in conservation of those water resources and more run-off resulting in increased flooding, as we have seen already occurring in California over the past few years.

Whether air quality or water scarcity, these issues will only be exacerbated by the fact that Utah is one of the fastest growing states in the nation. More people place demands for more housing, and a recent study already suggests the housing supply is short by thousands of units and already places over 40,000 low-income renters at risk for housing instability due to rapidly increasing rent and home prices (Wood and Becker 2023). This is particularly true for older adults on fixed incomes, where increases in rent and/or property taxes exceed any potential cost of living increase. It is staggering to consider that people aged 65 and older are the fastest growing demographic group experiencing homelessness (Culhane et al. 2019). Not surprisingly, this skews significantly toward underrepresented groups (Kushel 2020). One can only imagine that with the impending fiscal challenges associated with both Medicare and Social Security facing insolvency over the next decade, a fundamental reconsideration of age-friendly communities is incumbent.

Age-Friendly Communities as Ecosystems

This is why the following volume is brilliant in both its timeliness as well as its bold rethinking of age-friendly communities as ecosystems, or more specifically, resilient ecosystems. Fulmer and Huang (this volume) articulate five sectors as part of age-friendly ecosystems: public health, health systems, cities and communities, employers and universities. As an ecosystem, these five sectors need to work synergistically to foster collective resilience, requiring adaptive capacity of the ecosystem to respond to threats and dangers and recover quickly. The global COVID scare of the early 2020s reflects this interdependency. Public health determined a course of action including limiting social contact to limit transmission, including shutting down the economy. The health system was overrun as demonstrated by tent hospitals and medical ships being brought to large urban areas. Cities and communities became ghost towns, with significant economic damage to hospitality industries. Employers wrestled with how to keep their businesses operating, and advantages skewed to professional services with their digital access and capabilities, and away from manual labor-dependent industries. Finally, universities were called upon to research and provide care, along with their educational mission, while facing all of the above challenges. All of this arising from one virus. In short, the system proved not particularly agile to adapt, and, because of this, we are still recovering across numerous sectors. On reflection, my strong inference suggests all sectors, but particularly behavioral public health, rested their response on the reasonable person theory: that when provided information, people will do the reasonable thing. That proved not to be the case, and studies document excess deaths resulting from COVID-19, including differential rates in excess deaths associated with political affiliation. Who would have thought?

Age-Friendly Health Systems

This volume simplifies the Fulmer and Huang framework of age-friendly ecosystems to health systems (by collapsing public health and health systems together), universities and neighborhoods. Fulmer and Huang offer a "5 Cs Framework" for age-friendly public health systems: connecting and convening, coordinating, collecting (and disseminating) data, communicating, complementing (and supplementing). Connecting and convening suggests the importance of integrated actions to address emerging threats or problems and leads naturally to the need to coordinate such efforts. Collecting data and communicating not only the data but analyses and resulting prioritizations and receiving regular feedback are essential. Finally, complementing suggests the need for supportive efforts across multiple domains and multiple actions to drive a result.

In terms of age-friendly health care, the World Health Organization has identified three principles: information, education, communication and training of staff;

healthcare management systems adapting to the special needs of aging adults; and the physical environment reflecting universal design principles. In response to the first principle, Fulmer and Huang briefly mention the 4 Ms: what Matters: Medication (age-friendly medications and dosing); Mentation, engaging practices focused on dementia, delirium and depression; and Mobility, a focus on safe, physical functional ability. These practices are shared in a toolkit available from the Institute for Healthcare Improvement (2019). Unfortunately, recent studies suggest a lack of awareness and implementation of these practices in primary, secondary and tertiary care (Tavares et al. 2021). This reflects that age-friendly health systems remain in the pre-paradigmatic stage, and reinforces the timeliness of this volume.

Age-Friendly Neighborhoods

Hong (this volume) presents a chapter emphasizing the importance of the voices of older persons in shaping the design of age-friendly neighborhoods. The chapter provides an easily digestible overview of the challenges and opportunities for age-friendly neighborhoods. Challenges may be summarized as the lack of available accessible, affordable housing. Housing is often inaccessible in a couple of dimensions: (1) in terms of those meeting universal design guidelines for physical accessibility; and (2) inaccessibility to needed services or amenities, such as groceries, healthcare or parks. These concerns are then often exacerbated by financial considerations with more affordable housing located in more remote geographic locations. In fact, Hong raises a critical consideration for the Intermountain West, that the challenge paradigm for achieving age-friendly communities may well lay in our rural communities, and particularly those whose majority populations are indigenous.

Concerns such as these are the subject of the insightful chapter by Greer and Edelman that makes clear that underlying the notion of age-friendly is the question: "Age-friendly for whom?" This chapter offers a brilliant take that age-friendly ecosystems, like all ecosystems, become more supportive and resilient when they are inclusive of and responsive to diversity. While ecosystems from a biological perspective consider abiotic and biotic dimensions, human landscapes need to add the cultural dimension as well (Ndubisi 2002). In our push for generalizability, many principles overlook the criticality of ecological validity: how actions really work and are perceived in the lived world. Here, Greer and Edelman adopt the imageable phrase "place-based disparities," as inclusive of both the bundled hypotheses found in the "zip code paradigm" and the assertion by Wallace (2021) that the greatest challenges for older adults do not stem from biological, but rather social and political processes. It is not surprising that in earlier work, Wallace and colleagues brilliantly intersected spatial and racial injustice (Caldwell et al. 2016), a point echoed here.

What I find intriguing is that Greer and Edelman appear to point a way forward, with an orientation to become more place-based in our approach to age-friendly ecosystems. In their words, "It is fundamentally important to consider the plethora of social axes that combine with physical environments and personal identities to create health outcomes over the life-course" (Greer and Edelman, this volume). This call reminds me of the Ecological Framework of Place (Diaz Moore 2014), which suggested four key themes to connecting environmental gerontology with developmental science theory: (1) the integration of levels of organization within the socioecological system, (2) social embeddedness, (3) temporality and (4) human agency. These themes undergird their desire for "longitudinal and cross-national studies that account for the temporal characteristics of place" (Greer and Edelman, this volume).

Age-Friendly Campuses

The Age-Friendly University (AFU) initiative discussed by Montepare and colleagues (this volume) snaps into focus the challenges identified by other volume contributors. Here, it is actually quite logical that institutions of higher education—often sharing goals of access and inclusion—operating in a demographic reality that their core constituency is now shrinking should of course be leaning into age-inclusive practices and markets. Yet, we see the pervasive impact of historic institutionalism to resist the ten principles for an age-friendly university. Almost all the chapters discuss the potent force of ageism in our socio-political decision-making, but here, Montepare and colleagues raise the critical issue of reframing, in general, and the Reframing Aging Initiative specifically. As I read through this volume, the importance of understanding that the fundamental structure of our demographics is forever changed and that we no longer will have population pyramids, but simply population towers, proves essential. As opposed to an ever-shrinking demographic, older adults constitute as much of society as minors; in fact, by 2034 there will be more US citizens 65+ than 18 and under (US Census 2023).

This demographic reality provides a societal imperative for universities to truly embrace the notion of age-inclusiveness. The ten principles for an Age-Friendly University (AFU) are a wonderful beginning and raise significant opportunities for institutions of higher education to further their mission by broadening their sense of inclusion. How may (must?) universities capitalize on and optimize the longevity dividend? In a very concrete way, principle 9, to engage actively with the university's own retired community, is to maximize the axiom at most universities "when you are a (mascot), you are a (mascot) for life." This portends reconsideration of the business model of education and raises the potential for educational savings accounts for life-long learning to perhaps membership or subscription models. Additionally, residential campuses may do well to consider shaping community life and residential models for older adults; so-called university-based retirement communities (UBRC), as advocated for by Montepare and colleagues (2019) elsewhere. For such UBRCs to be successful, Smith and colleagues (2014) identified seven criteria: (1) proximity, to enable mental stimulation, physical activation and familiarity; (2) bi-directional programming; (3) continuing-care component, to further safety and continuity; (4) a financial link, to do the same; (5) minimum 10 percent alumni, to further identity; (6) integrated transportation; and (7) facilitating activity. Sought is the same level of integration for these UBRCs as there is for student housing, which stands to reason, as they are simply another key demographic group of an enlarged sense of community.

Looking Forward

It is clear that each chapter in this volume identifies critical advances in the age-friendliness of communities but also offers significant gaps in our current approach to place-making for an unquestionably aging society. The issues raised become magnified in the challenging environment of the Intermountain West with its water scarcity, air quality issues, unsustainable patterns of suburban development and the climate crisis exacerbating all of these with each passing year. Whether at the scale of climate, policy, community or buildings, it is quite clear that the Intermountain West faces persistently growing drivers of needed change and experimentation in the coming decade. Age-friendly communities present a wicked problem to society; "a problem that is difficult or impossible to solve because of incomplete and contradictory data, deeply-entangled relationships, and changing requirements that are often difficult to recognize or tease apart" (Diaz Moore 2017). Yet the felicitous concept of age-friendly ecosystem may provide a north star, not as to the solutions themselves, but a direction to potentially get there.

If we truly conceive of a resilient age-friendly ecosystem, then we might be wise to understand what are the characteristics of a resilient ecology. Scown and colleagues (2023) identify nine factors of ecological resilience: (bio)diversity, spatial and temporal variability, within-scale and cross-scale feedbacks, production of services at multiple scales, fast or tight versus slow variables, connectivity, governance, social capital and feedbacks amongst governance organizations and ecological change.

The concept of diversity is sprinkled throughout this volume, whether in terms of intersectionality or the need for a range of responses to meet the heterogeneous aging experience. Spatial and temporality variability are precise challenges to our exclusionary zoning practices that segregate care facilities from residential neighborhoods and 8am–5pm work areas from bedroom communities. Arguably the main theme of the volume is the notion of within-scale and cross-scale feedbacks, such as do our policies facilitate the heterogeneity in the built environment that is clearly essential to achieve age-friendly communities? Production of services at multiple scales is a complex concept but perhaps best exemplified in terms of transportation. One can think of last-mile transportation closest to one's residence, but do mobility networks connect and extend appropriately, or do they arbitrarily end at, say, county lines? The speed of variables is a fascinating concept. As an example, long variables in terms of age-friendly campuses such as building a retirement community may take years, while incorporating universal design in course websites can be implemented quickly as a short variable if there is the will. Connectivity is referenced heavily in terms of independent mobility, but is also a critical theme discussed in terms of age-friendly health systems. Simple transferability of health data between service systems is critical for more efficacious care. Arguably this also highlights the concepts of governance (what is allowable by policy?) and feedback amongst governance organizations. Lastly, social capital and its connection to age-friendly communities is a ubiquitous theme for healthy aging in the gerontological literature (c.f., Diaz Moore et al. 2019; Scharlach and Diaz Moore 2016).

These nine concepts provide rich, intellectual fodder to consider design principles for an age-friendly ecosystem. This volume inspires the following as an initial set, demanding revisitation and refinement, but hopefully illustrative of the inspiration provided herein. Age-friendly ecosystems need to:

- Promote diversity in environmental, financial, policy and care response across all three levels of the system in order to allow the broadest range of individuals to thrive.
- Foster spatial and temporal variability in its provision of environments, care and services.
- Optimize within-scale and cross-scale feedback and redundancy of responses desired to forward critical goals of healthy aging.
- Produce and foster responsive services at each level of the ecosystem.
- Make decisions with fidelity to the speed of response expected from the change to the system.
- Maximize the connectivity and integration between systems.
- Align policy responses at all levels of governance.
- Orient all care, policy and environmental interventions to promote social connectedness.
- Foster double-loop learning with meaningful feedback from older adults, their allies, advocates and providers in all organizations.

This is the type of creativity inspired by the chapters to follow. When reviewed, these principles would be equally useful in addressing the macro-issues confronting the Intermountain West. A useful foundational question over the coming decades may well be "How do we create a more resilient age-friendly ecosystem that enhances the adaptive capacity of the regional ecology itself?" Our ecology is fragile and threatened by the drivers of human suburban development and climate change resulting from our twentieth-century approach to settlement for the baby boom generation. But the population pyramid demographic assumed by the model no longer exists. A new age distribution for society is on the horizon, demanding complete rethinking of how we design our communities. It may well be that creating age-friendly ecosystems holds the key to understanding interventions that may both facilitate human thriving and ecological flourishing.

University of Utah
Salt Lake City, UT, USA

Keith Diaz Moore

References

Caldwell, J.T., C.L. Ford, S.P. Wallace, M.C. Wang, and L.M. Takahashi. 2016. Intersection of Living in a Rural Versus Urban Area and Race/Ethnicity in Explaining Access to Health Care in the United States. *American Journal of Public Health* 106 (8): 1463–1469.

Culhane, D., D. Treglia, T. Byrne, S. Metraux, R. Kuhn, K. Doran, E. Johns, and M. Schretzman. 2019. *The Emerging Crisis of Aged Homelessness*. Philadelphia: Actionable Intelligence for Social Policy at the University of Pennsylvania.

Diaz Moore, K. 2014. An Ecological Framework of Place: Situating Environmental Gerontology Within a Life Course Perspective. *The International Journal of Aging and Human Development* 79 (3): 183–209.

Diaz Moore, K. 2017. *Lecture on Wicked Problems in the Class DES 2615: Introduction to Design Thinking*. University of Utah.

Diaz Moore, K., Garcia, I., and J. Kim. 2019. Healthy Places and the Social Life of Older Adults. In *Social Isolation of Older Adults*, ed. L. Kaye, and C. Singer. New York: Springer.

Diaz Moore, K., E. Greenfield, and A. Scharlach. 2017. Healthy Aging and Its Implications for Public Health: Healthy Communities. In *Aging, Place and Health: A Global Perspective*, ed. W. Satariano and M. Maus. Sudbury: Jones & Bartlett.

Errigo, I. M., B. W. Abbott, D. L. Mendoza, L. Mitchell, S. S. Sayedi, J. Glenn, K. E. Kelly, J. D. Beard, S. Bratsman, T. Carter, R. A. Chaney, A. Follett, A. Freeman, R. J. Frei, M. Greenhalgh, H. A. Holmes, P. D. Howe, J. D. Johnston, L. Lange, R. Martin, A. Stacey, T. Tran, and D. Wilson. 2020. Human Health and Economic Costs of Air Pollution in Utah: An Expert Assessment. *Atmosphere* 11 (11): 1238.

Golant, S. M. 2015. Residential Normalcy and the Enriched Coping Repertoires of Successfully Aging Older Adults. *The Gerontologist* 55 (1): 70–82.

Greenfield, E. A., and T. Buffel. 2022. Age-Friendly Cities and Communities: Research to Strengthen Policy and Practice. *Journal of Aging & Social Policy* 34 (2): 161–174.

Healy, J. 2023. A Puzzle in Arizona's Boom Towns: How to Keep Growing with Less Water. *The New York Times*. https://www.nytimes.com/2023/06/09/us/arizona-water-development-desert.html.

Institute for Healthcare Improvement. 2019. "What matters" to Older Adults? A Toolkit for Health Systems to Design Better Care with Older Adults. *Age-Friendly Health Systems*. https://www.ihi.org/Engage/Initiatives/Age-Friendly-Health-Systems/Documents/IHI_Age_Friendly_What_Matters_to_Older_Adults_Toolkit.pdf. Accessed 4 Sep 2023.

Khatri, K. B., C. Strong, A. K. Kochanski, S. Burian, C. Miller, and C. Hasenyager. 2018. Water Resources Criticality Due to Future Climate Change and Population Growth: Case of River Basins in Utah, USA. *Journal of Water Resources Planning and Management* 144 (8): 04018041.

Kushel, M. 2020. Homelessness Among Older Adults: An Emerging Crisis. *Generations* 44 (2): 1–7.

LaPlante, J., and B. McCann. 2008. Complete Streets: We Can Get There from Here. *ITE Journal* 78 (5): 24.

Lui, C. W., J. A. Everingham, J. Warburton, M. Cuthill, and H. Bartlett. 2009. What Makes a Community Age-Friendly: A Review of International Literature. *Australasian Journal on Ageing* 28: 116–121. https://doi.org/10.1111/j.1741-6612.2009.00355.x

Montepare, J. M., K. S. Farah, A. Doyle, and J. Dixon. 2019. Becoming an Age-Friendly University (AFU): Integrating a Retirement Community on Campus. *Gerontology & Geriatrics Education* 40 (2): 179–193.

Ndubisi, F. 2002. *Ecological Planning: A Historical and Comparative Synthesis*. JHU Press.

Oberlink, M. R. 2008. *Opportunities for Creating Livable Communities*. Washington: AARP, Public Policy Institute.

Osborne, M. 2023. Drying Great Salt Lake Could Expose Millions to Toxic Arsenic-laced Dust. *Smithsonian Magazine*. https://www.smithsonianmag.com/smart-news/drying-great-salt-lake-could-expose-millions-to-toxic-arsenic-laced-dust-180981439/.

Pynoos, J., C. Cicero, and C. M. Nishita. 2010. New Challenges and Growing Trends in Senior Housing. In *The New Politics of Old Age Policy*, ed. R. B. Hudson, 2nd edition, p. Baltimore: Johns Hopkins University Press.

Scharlach, A., and K. Diaz Moore. 2016. Aging-in-Place. In *Handbook of Theories of Aging*, ed. V. Bengston, and R. Setterston, 3rd edition. New York: Springer.

Scown, M. W., R. K. Craig, C. R. Allen, L. Gunderson, D. G. Angeler, J. H. Garcia, and A. Garmestani. 2023. Towards a Global Sustainable Development Agenda Built on Social–Ecological Resilience. *Global Sustainability* 6: e8.

Smith, E. K., E. K. Rozek, and K. D Moore. 2014. Creating SPOTs for Successful Aging: Strengthening the Case for Developing University-Based Retirement Communities Using Social-Physical Place Over Time Theory. *Journal of Housing for the Elderly* 28 (1): 21–40.

Tavares, J., G. Santinha, and N. P. Rocha. 2021. Age-Friendly Health Care: A Systematic Review. *Healthcare* 9 (1): 83. https://doi.org/10.3390/healthcare9010083.

US Census. 2023. Older People Projected to Outnumber Children for First Time in U.S. History. Retrieved September 4, 2023 from https://www.census.gov/newsroom/press-releases/2018/cb18-41-population-projections.html#:~:text="By%202034%20(previously%202035),decade%20for%20the%20U.S.%20population

Village Movement. n.d. *Home – Village to Village Network, Inc.* https://www.vtvnetwork.org/. Accessed 1 Nov 2023.

Wood, J., and M. Becker. 2023. *A Comparison of State-Funded Affordable Housing Programs*. Salt Lake City: The Gardner Policy Institute. https://gardner.utah.edu/wp-content/uploads/HousingPoliciesRep-Apr2023.pdf?x71849

World Health Organization. 2007. *Global Age-Friendly Cities: A Guide*. World Health Organization.

Preface

People live longer and healthier than ever before but we live in places that were designed for significantly shorter lifespans. How can the environments where we live transform as rapidly as our aging population, and create age-friendly futures?

Age-friendliness has grown from an idea into a social movement that recognizes the diversity of older adults, and integrates research, policy, programming and design. The pressures of rapid aging, systemic ageism and a growing disparity of resources create an urgent need to rethink how we achieve equity in aging through design of places and practices.

This book examines age-friendliness within the framework of age-friendly ecosystems, and from a place-based approach, considering anchor institutions of neighborhoods, campuses and health environments as sites uniquely positioned to catalyze age equity and inclusivity.

Content for this book draws from a symposium which editors created in 2022, Age-Friendly Communities as Platforms for Equity, Health & Wellness. Contributing authors build upon the content shared through the symposium in order to examine how neighborhoods, campuses and health environments are uniquely poised to support equity and to extend reach to historically marginalized populations of older adults. Ideas and experiences that were presented by national experts in aging are presented through a place-based approach, as are "real-world" experiences and narratives shared by older adults, students, community stakeholders and faculty researchers who participated in the symposium. Graphic notes from the symposium are illustrated in Figs. 1, 2, 3, 4, and 5.

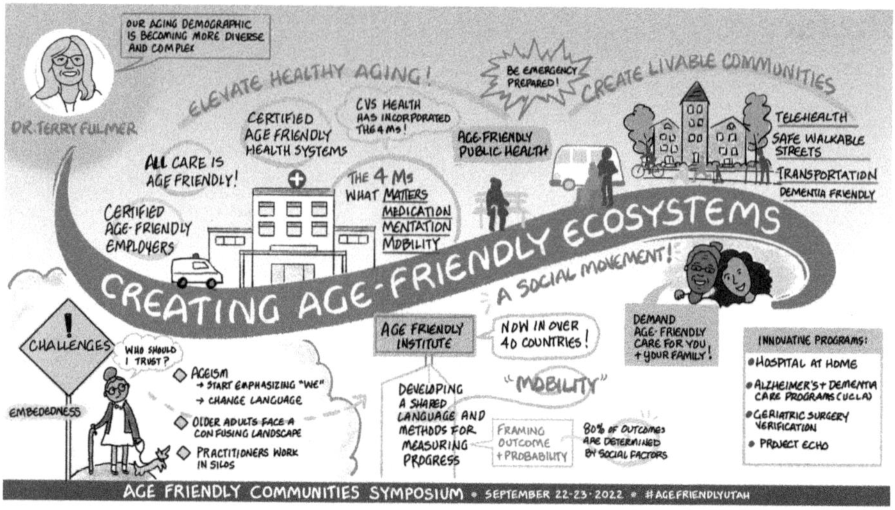

Fig. 1 Age-friendly ecosystems: age-friendly communities symposium graphic notes. (Credit: Alece Birnbach)

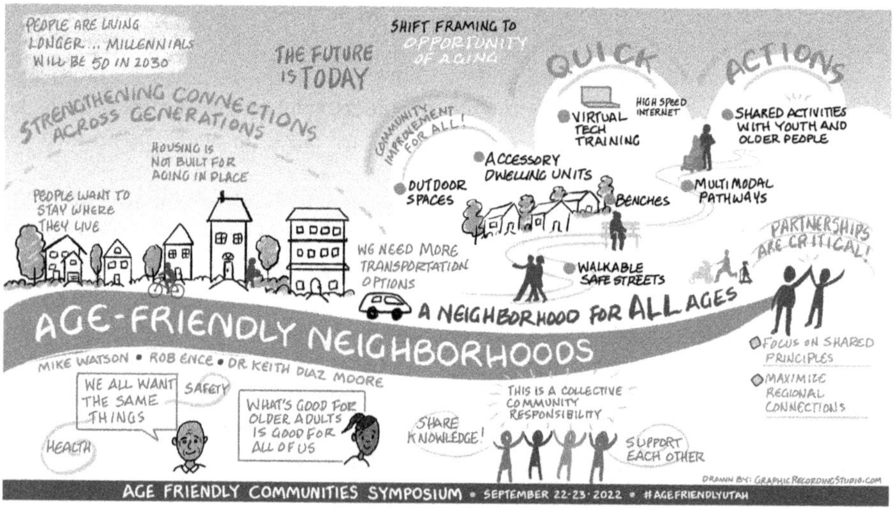

Fig. 2 Age-friendly neighborhoods: age-friendly communities symposium graphic notes. (Credit: Alece Birnbach)

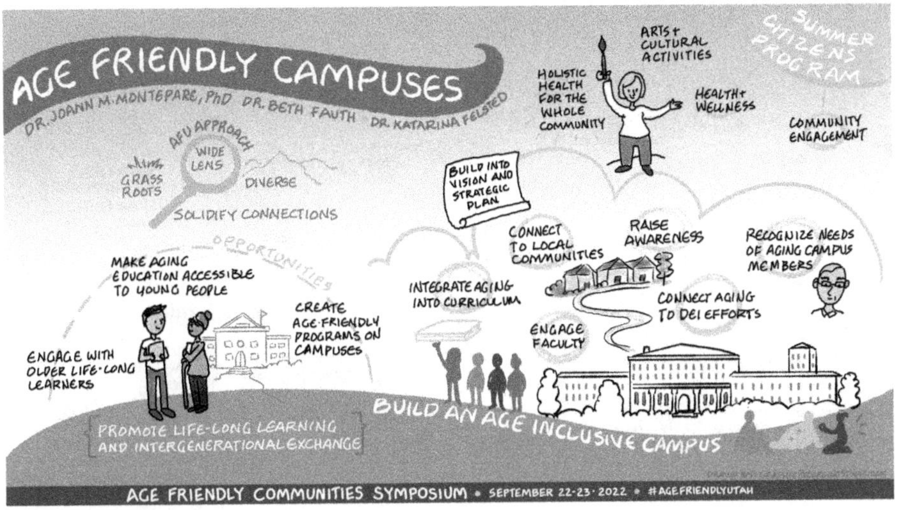
AGE FRIENDLY CAMPUSES
DR. JOANN M. MONTEPARE, PhD DR. BETH FAUTH DR. KATARINA FELSTED
AFU APPROACH
WIDE LENS
GRASS ROOTS
DIVERSE
SOLIDIFY CONNECTIONS
OPPORTUNITIES
MAKE AGING EDUCATION ACCESSIBLE TO YOUNG PEOPLE
CREATE AGE-FRIENDLY PROGRAMS ON CAMPUSES
ENGAGE WITH OLDER LIFE-LONG LEARNERS
PROMOTE LIFE-LONG LEARNING AND INTERGENERATIONAL EXCHANGE
BUILD INTO VISION AND STRATEGIC PLAN
HOLISTIC HEALTH FOR THE WHOLE COMMUNITY
ARTS + CULTURAL ACTIVITIES
HEALTH + WELLNESS
SUMMER CITIZENS PROGRAM
COMMUNITY ENGAGEMENT
CONNECT TO LOCAL COMMUNITIES
RAISE AWARENESS
RECOGNIZE NEEDS OF AGING CAMPUS MEMBERS
INTEGRATE AGING INTO CURRICULUM
CONNECT AGING TO DEI EFFORTS
ENGAGE FACULTY
BUILD AN AGE INCLUSIVE CAMPUS
AGE FRIENDLY COMMUNITIES SYMPOSIUM • SEPTEMBER 22-23-2022 • #AGEFRIENDLYUTAH

Fig. 3 Age-friendly campuses: age-friendly communities symposium graphic notes. (Credit: Alece Birnbach)

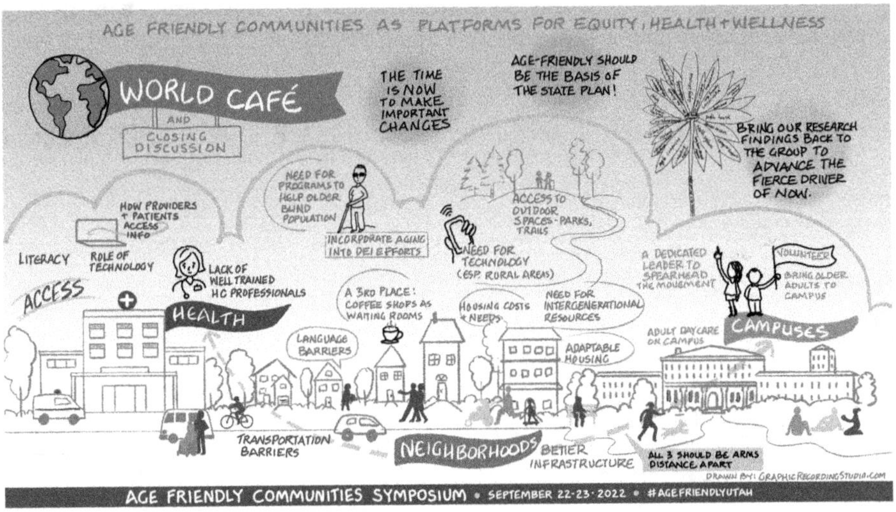

Fig. 5 Age-friendly voices: world café; age-friendly communities symposium graphic notes. (Credit: Alece Birnbach)

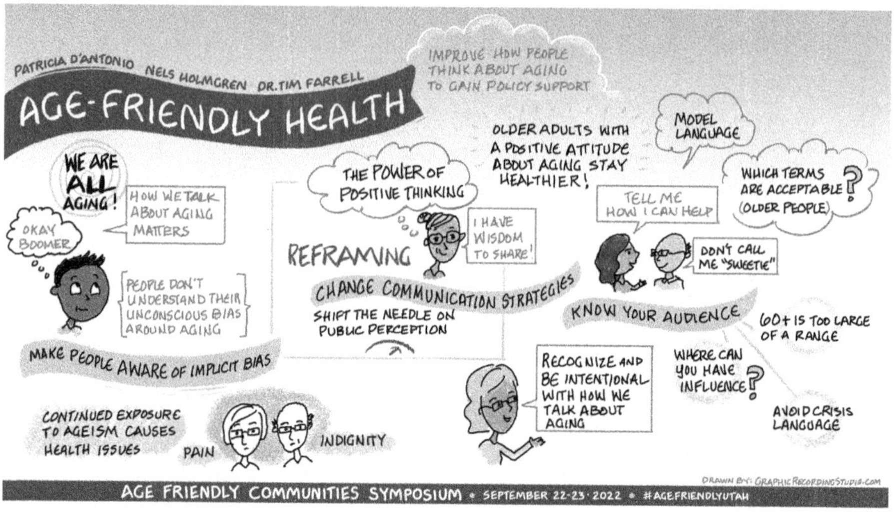
PATRICIA D'ANTONIO
NELS HOLMGREN
DR. TIM FARRELL
AGE-FRIENDLY HEALTH
IMPROVE HOW PEOPLE THINK ABOUT AGING TO GAIN POLICY SUPPORT
OLDER ADULTS WITH A POSITIVE ATTITUDE ABOUT AGING STAY HEALTHIER!
MODEL LANGUAGE
WHICH TERMS ARE ACCEPTABLE? (OLDER PEOPLE)
WE ARE ALL AGING!
HOW WE TALK ABOUT AGING MATTERS
OKAY BOOMER
THE POWER OF POSITIVE THINKING
I HAVE WISDOM TO SHARE!
TELL ME HOW I CAN HELP
DON'T CALL ME "SWEETIE"
REFRAMING
PEOPLE DON'T UNDERSTAND THEIR UNCONSCIOUS BIAS AROUND AGING
CHANGE COMMUNICATION STRATEGIES
SHIFT THE NEEDLE ON PUBLIC PERCEPTION
KNOW YOUR AUDIENCE
60+ IS TOO LARGE OF A RANGE
MAKE PEOPLE AWARE OF IMPLICIT BIAS
RECOGNIZE AND BE INTENTIONAL WITH HOW WE TALK ABOUT AGING
WHERE CAN YOU HAVE INFLUENCE?
AVOID CRISIS LANGUAGE
CONTINUED EXPOSURE TO AGEISM CAUSES HEALTH ISSUES
PAIN
INDIGNITY
DRAWN BY: GRAPHICRECORDINGSTUDIO.COM
AGE FRIENDLY COMMUNITIES SYMPOSIUM • SEPTEMBER 22-23 · 2022 • #AGEFRIENDLYUTAH

Fig. 4 Age-friendly health: age-friendly communities symposium graphic notes. (Credit: Alece Birnbach)

Collectively, the voices in this book create a lens for empowering age-friendly ecosystems as environments for equitable aging by design.

Salt Lake City, UT, USA

Valerie Chang Greer
Linda S. Edelman

Acknowledgments

The work of creating age-friendly places requires action and collaboration among many fields. We are honored to have contributions to this book from an interdisciplinary team of experts, representing fields of health, policy, education, planning and design. Our heartfelt gratitude goes to the College of Architecture and Planning at the University of Utah, and the Utah Geriatric Education Consortium for sponsorship and unwavering support of the symposium and this book. Thank you to Dr. Terry Fulmer whose generosity contributed to the ability to engage students in the symposium, and to Ashley Cadiz whose work in organizing the Koi Pond Student Ideas Competition provided an avenue for students to engage.

We are grateful for the support of an outstanding Advisory Board and a Student Advisory Committee. Thank you to Board Members and students for invaluable guidance and dedication in creating the symposium, and supporting the proposal for this book. We are grateful for the talent and beautiful work that Alece Birnbach contributed to in creating graphic notes for the symposium. Lastly, we thank the participants who contributed to the symposium and shared their perspectives and work. We hope the community of voices shared through this book provides insight, inspiration and resources impactful to your work.

About the Book/Conference

The goal of our symposium and this book is to promote aging well across the life span. Contemporary social, environmental and health issues, compounded with the rapidly aging population and the prevalence of ageism, point to a need for new scholarship and action focused on age-friendly communities as they shape socio-environmental determinants of health and wellness. Design has a significant role to play in shaping how intersectional characteristics of people integrate with multiple dimensions of place, and shape experiences of aging in years to come.

We build upon the framework of age-friendly ecosystems as a collective design project, with focus on how age-friendly neighborhoods, campuses and health environments can empower choice, equity and positive health outcomes in the context of contemporary and future challenges. Challenges that are specific to the Intermountain West are considered as this region hosts a flagship of social, health and environmental issues including extreme population growth, environmental degradation and lack of affordability. The symposium and this book aim to bring forth scholarship, educational materials and advocacy that will advance the understanding, development and social impact of age friendly communities.

Contents

About the Editors

Valerie Chang Greer, AIA, LEED AP, is an Assistant Professor at the University of Utah College of Architecture + Planning and an architect with experience designing healthcare facilities, campuses and housing. Greer is Director of Graduate Studies in the School of Architecture and co-Director of the Healthy Aging Resilient Places (HARP) Lab at the University of Utah. Her research utilizes participatory community engagement and co-creation methods to explore the impact of built environments on health and wellness. Greer teaches design studios and professional practice at the undergraduate and graduate levels.

Linda S. Edelman, PhD, RN, is a Professor in the University of Utah College of Nursing. Her research focus is rural aging and improving older adult care transitions through interprofessional education and community-based research. Dr. Edelman leads the Utah Geriatric Education Consortium (UGEC), an interprofessional HRSA-funded workforce development grant focusing on improving the life and care of older adults through age-friendly care. The UGEC partners with U Health's Age-Friendly Health Systems initiative and with long-term services and supports organizations across Utah to implement the "4Ms" framework.

Contributors

Lauren Marshall Bowen, PhD, Department of English, College of Liberal Arts, Gerontology Department and Institute, Manning College of Nursing and Health Sciences, University of Massachusetts Boston, Boston, MA, USA

Sarah L. Canham, PhD, College of Social Work, University Health Interprofessional Education Program, Healthy Aging and Resilient Places Lab, The University of Utah, Salt Lake City, UT, USA

Valerie Chang Greer, AIA, LEED AP, NOMA, College of Architecture and Planning, Graduate Studies, School of Architecture, Healthy Aging and Resilient Places Lab, The University of Utah, Salt Lake City, UT, USA

Patricia M. D'Antonio, BSPharm, MS, MBA, BCGP, Policy and Professional Affairs, Gerontological Society of America, Washington, DC, USA

National Center to Reframe Aging, Washington, DC, USA

Linda S. Edelman, RN, PhD, FGSA, FAAN, College of Nursing, Hartford Center of Geriatric Nursing Excellence, Utah Geriatric Education Consortium (UGEC), Utah Rural Opioid Consortium Collaborative Care Model (UROHC-CCM), The University of Utah, Salt Lake City, UT, USA

Kimberly S. Farah, PhD, School of Health Sciences, Lasell University, Newton, MA, USA

Timothy W. Farrell, MD, AGSF, Division of Geriatrics, Spencer Fox Eccles School of Medicine, VA SLC Geriatric Research, Education, and Clinical Center, University of Utah Academy of Health Science Educators, The University of Utah, Salt Lake City, UT, USA

Katarina Friberg-Felsted, PhD, FAGHE, Gerontology Interdisciplinary Program, College of Nursing, The University of Utah, Salt Lake City, UT, USA

Terry Fulmer, PhD, RN, FAAN, The John A. Hartford Foundation, New York, NY, USA

Andy Hong, PhD, Healthy Aging and Resilient Places Lab, Department of City and Metropolitan Planning, College of Architecture + Planning, The University of Utah, Salt Lake City, UT, USA

Jessica Huang The John A. Hartford Foundation, New York, NY, USA

Columbia University Mailman School of Public Health, New York, NY, USA

Joann M. Montepare, PhD, Rosemary B. Fuss Center for Research on Aging and Intergenerational Studies, Lasell University, Newton, MA, USA

Nina M. Silverstein, PhD, Gerontology Department and Institute, Manning College of Nursing and Health Sciences, University of Massachusetts Boston, Boston, MA, USA

Susan K. Whitbourne, PhD, Department of Psychological and Brain Sciences; Gerontology Department and Institute, Manning College of Nursing and Health Sciences, University of Massachusetts Amherst, Boston, Boston, MA, USA

Department of Gerontology, John W. McCormack Graduate School of Policy & Global Studies, University of Massachusetts Boston, Boston, MA, USA

Chapter 1
Creating an Age-Friendly Environment Across the Ecosystem

Terry Fulmer and Jessica Huang

Introduction

Across the world, people are aging. In 2020, 1 billion people were aged 60 or older, and by 2050 that number will double to 2.1 billion (*Aging and Health* 2022). A longer life can lead to an array of benefits for older adults and society. Additional years offer the chance to pursue new activities, build social relationships, and contribute to one's family and the community. However, the opportunity to fully utilize this new time is contingent upon maintaining good health and good function. The physical and social environment plays a substantial role in the long-term trajectory of healthy aging, but many older adults are finding it difficult to maintain healthy behaviors due to a lack of an age-friendly infrastructure to support older adults as they age (Fulmer et al. 2020). Older adults are more likely to have a health profile that is extremely complex with multiple chronic conditions, and, at times, instructions from their medical providers that conflict from team to team. This puts them at risk for disproportionate harm with higher rates of health-related harm and lack of coordinated care, as well as extremely poor preparation for disasters, as in the case of Hurricane Katrina and more recently the COVID-19 pandemic (Durant Jr 2011; Ouslander and Grabowski 2020). This chapter explores the implementation of age-friendly ecosystems and the benefits that can be reaped by contributing to an age-friendly global movement.

T. Fulmer (✉)
The John A. Hartford Foundation, New York, NY, USA
e-mail: Terry.Fulmer@johnahartford.org

J. Huang
The John A. Hartford Foundation, New York, NY, USA

Columbia University Mailman School of Public Health, New York, NY, USA
e-mail: Jessica.Huang@johnahartford.org

V. Chang Greer, L. S. Edelman (eds.), *Age-Friendly Ecosystems*, SpringerBriefs in Public Health, https://doi.org/10.1007/978-3-031-68361-9_1

The Policy Lever

From a policymaker standpoint, it is of the utmost importance to support policy that advances the health and well-being of older adults. Many older adults' additional years are characterized by a decline in physical, cognitive, and mental health, which can have negative implications for older adults, their families, and broader society. Out-of-pocket healthcare expenditures are significant for this age group, 20 percent of older Americans face out-of-pocket healthcare costs over $2000, leading to postponed or forgone care (Jacobson et al. 2021). These costs also create a payer incentive to maximize necessary and efficient high-quality care. Skipped or delayed care can lead to increases in chronic and costly conditions. In 2021, the average Medicare per person spending reached over $15,000, a number only expected to increase with an aging population (2022). With this momentous change in the population demographic, it is essential to adapt and innovate in order to enrich the lives of this growing sector of our community, ensure quality care, and prevent healthcare-induced harm. This line of thinking is giving rise to the age-friendly ecosystem framework.

What Is an Age-Friendly Ecosystem?

Age-friendly is defined as environments that promote access to options, key services, and opportunities for people of all ages and that promote the inclusion and participation of older adults in all aspects of life (Kalache et al. 2004) (Fig. 1.1). The age-friendly movement has been underway for decades, but it gained traction when the World Health Organization (WHO) endorsed the Vienna International Plan of Action on Aging (Fulmer et al. 2020). Extensive progress has been made in the different sectors that have taken on the call for "age-friendly," such as age-friendly cities; however, a multi-sector initiative is imperative to accelerate the global age-friendly vision. Experts agree that cross-sector collaboration will bring more impactful, long-term improvements (Dash et al. 2022). Age-friendly practitioners are already doing transformational work in six existing frameworks (The John A. Hartford Foundation, n.d.):

1. Cities, communities, and State.
2. Education and research.
3. Healthcare systems.
4. Public health.
5. Workplaces.
6. Home and community-based services.

Age-friendly ecosystems can bolster this work by providing a unified approach to develop a shared understanding of what it means to be age-friendly across all settings and help provide a framework for cross-sector collaboration with measurable impact.

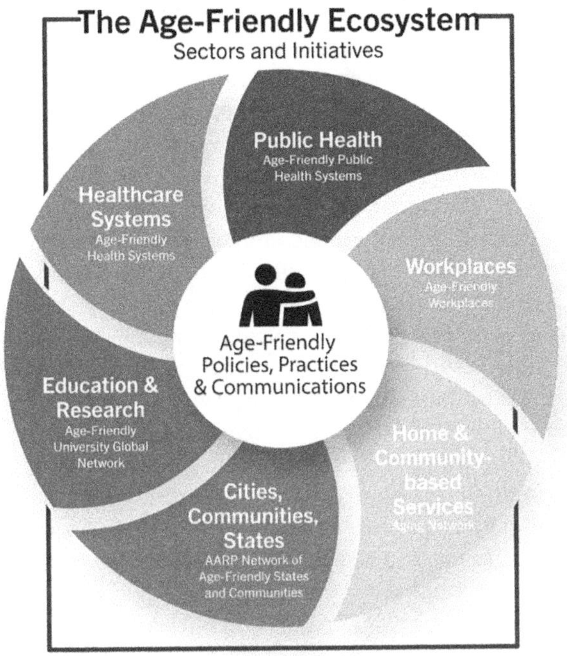

Fig. 1.1 Age-friendly ecosystem graphic. (The John A. Hartford Foundation n.d.)

Why Is It Important?

Numerous evidence-based models are meant to improve the lives of older adults, but many are not reliably applied, due to a lack of successful dissemination of information to the providers who can offer them and the consumers who may benefit. Examples include the acute care for the elderly (ACE) unit model, which requires dedicated clinical space and staff, or the Alzheimer's and Dementia Care Program (ADCP), which requires advanced practice nurses who are experts in dementia care (Landefeld et al. 1995; Reuben et al. 2022). Additional challenges include difficulty scaling programs, reproducing age-friendly care in health systems with fewer resources, and challenges translating age-friendly practices across different care settings. The age-friendly ecosystem movement works to ensure that all care is equitable and accessible by implementing evidence-based practices, such as the 4Ms, and is consistent with "What Matters" to the older adult and their family. By also bringing together multiple sectors, it creates a more unified and cohesive approach to maximize beneficial impact. There is a growing body of literature that is improving on the way the "What Matters" M is measured, and the Veterans Administration is taking a solid lead in developing measures of system-level effects across the 4Ms and improving the way they tie together (Burke et al. 2022).

How to Create an Age-Friendly Ecosystem?

There is increasing global interest and activity to create and disseminate elements of the age-friendly ecosystem. Various cities and countries have taken different approaches to achieve this goal. Some notable examples of successful implementation include Brussels, Manchester, and Japan (Aung et al. 2020; Buffel et al. 2014). Each locale has adopted a unique approach tailored to its communities, but regardless there is a consistent, concerted, and collaborative effort from each of the five sectors of age-friendly ecosystems: public health, health systems, cities and communities, employers, and universities. Due to the extent of stakeholders involved, a "national response" is needed to drive forward the movement (De Biasi et al. 2020).

In the United States, there is a focus on encouraging more collaboration between and among the public health spheres and aging sectors. Trust for America's Health's (TFAH) "Age-Friendly Public Health Systems (AFPHS)" initiative provides an example of successful scaling in the public health sphere (De Biasi et al. 2020; Mate et al. 2021). The program is focused on highlighting healthy aging as a core function of public health by partnering with state and local health departments. Their work across various US states has resulted in improved outcomes and greatly contributed to the goal of eventually achieving an age-friendly public health system. TFAH developed a framework to test and implement age-friendly public health practices in several States, which contributed to the expansion of the AFPHS Initiative.

In 2022, TFAH updated its framework to include six key components, known as the 6Cs. The updated 6C framework provides a blueprint for developing the age-friendly public health system (Wolfe and Gracia 2023). The 6Cs, outlined in Table 1.1, provide clear action items for public health departments and other stakeholders to create age-friendly public health systems that support the health and well-being of older adults.

Table 1.1 The age-friendly public health systems 6C framework

Component	Description
Creating	Creating and leading policy, systems, and environmental changes to improve older adult health and well-being
Connecting	Connecting and convening multi-sector stakeholders to address the health and social needs of older adults through collective impact approaches focused on the social determinants of health
Coordinating	Coordinating existing supports and services to help older adults, families, and caregivers navigate and access services and supports, avoid duplication, and promote an integrated system of care
Collecting	Collecting, analyzing, and translating relevant and robust data on older adults to identify the needs and assets of a community and inform the development of interventions through community-wide assessment
Communicating	Communicating important public health information to promote and support older adult health and well-being, including conducting and disseminating research findings and emerging and best practices to support healthy aging
Complementing	Complementing existing health-promoting programs to ensure that they are adequately meeting the needs of older adults

Source: Reprinted from Wolfe and Gracia (2023). https://doi.org/10.3390/geriatrics8030063,

Factors leading to the success of model spread and scale include education, data collection, data monitoring, and collaboration. Before any formal initiatives can be initiated, those involved need to understand the "why" behind any proposed change; how they will feel supported in the work, what data will need to be collected, and how to use the plan-do-study-act cycle to monitor change and adjust practice accordingly (Langley et al. 2009). Further, determining community needs among and between the ecosystem components helps formulate the goals for each stakeholder so that efforts can be coordinated. Coordinating and measuring the efficacy of these programs ensures positive change is underway and helps answer the "why" for those involved.

Amid increased urbanization, another important area of work gaining traction is building livable communities, which are an indispensable part of creating an age-friendly ecosystem (AFE) (Fitzgerald and Caro 2014). Characteristics of age-friendly communities (AFC) include safe, walkable streets, transportation options, outdoor spaces, social participation, and community support and health services (Kim et al. 2022). An additional aspect of building these communities is ensuring they are dementia-friendly by cultivating a safe, respectful, and informed setting that supports building a high-quality life (Hung et al., 2021).

An important aspect of developing AFCs is to consider the culture of the population you are working with (Chao and Huang 2016). Taiwan's experience with AFCs provides an example of the importance of a culturally aligned initiative. Taiwan was one of the first Asian countries that began to promote AFCs following WHO's endorsement of the movement. They utilized the framework WHO provided, but differences in cultural values limited the paradigm's ability to be integrated as successfully as in Western communities. A culturally tailored AFC model may be more beneficial in aiding the global AFE movement.

Ageism

The ecosystem analysis has done much to help identify what some have called "internalized ageism," when an older adult begins to believe the limitations that are assigned to them as the default for how they behave and the lifestyles they choose. Further, this internalized ageism can lead to poor choices in health behaviors and treatment modalities. For example, an older person can believe that they are too old to stop smoking or that a hip replacement will not be helpful.

Ageism has been defined as prejudice or discrimination on the grounds of a person's age (Butler 1975). Ageism is rampant in the United States and has a negative impact on health and well-being. Older people are referred to as "they" and "the other" instead of "us" and "we." The Reframing Institute in Washington DC is doing much to help develop language that is respectful and inclusive that can be substituted for the ageist language we currently see in our daily greeting cards as well as on television and in the skits of comedians (Busso et al. 2018). More seriously, ageism is dangerous when the context becomes we versus them, young versus old, and who should get governmental support. The term "greedy geezers" is still prevalent, and older people are at times asked to step aside to make way for younger people instead of figuring out how the collective of society is where we will gain strength and positive outcomes in policies and practices. Ageism can be even more detrimental as it applies to older adults who are diverse. The data are clear that race and ethnicity play a serious role in negative patient experiences and disparate health outcomes (Hayes-Larson et al. 2021).

AFE and Diversity, Equity, and Inclusion

Being an older adult and identifying with a minority group can increase the risk of poor health outcomes due to the reduced likelihood of receiving quality health care compared to White counterparts (Du and Xu 2016). Many minority older adults are hesitant to seek out care due to perceived racism from providers. This tendency to delay care fuels health disparities (Rhee et al. 2019). COVID-19 highlighted the disparate health outcomes experienced by minority older adults, particularly among older Black adults who experienced higher rates of morbidity and mortality (Chatters et al. 2020). Institutionalized racist and ageist practices across sectors, such as healthcare systems and policies, magnified social vulnerabilities and left many older Black adults increasingly susceptible to health risks. All of us need to work across the ecosystem to eradicate ageism and race-based inequities (Korte et al. 2022).

Age-Friendly Universities

Recent work has proposed age-friendly universities (AFU) as a crucial initiative to combat ageism (Montepare and Brown 2022). This work is especially necessary in the wake of COVID-19, which has exacerbated ageist views through skewed media discourse that othered older adults by disproportionately emphasizing the need for isolation due to older adults' vulnerability. AFUs could mitigate ageism by allowing older adults to participate in higher education for their own personal and professional fulfillment, as well as incorporate education and research on aging for younger students. This will facilitate intergenerational exchange, which according to Levy's Positive Education about Aging and Contact Experiences (PEACE) can break down negative stereotypes and build more intergenerational camaraderie (Levy 2018).

Age-Friendly Health Systems as a Component of the Ecosystem

The John A. Hartford Foundation (JAHF) and the Institute for Healthcare Improvement (IHI), in partnership with the American Hospital Association (AHA), and the Catholic Health Association (CHA), have formed a collaboration that ensures a coordinated way forward so that older adults across the United States have safe and evidence-based care in alignment with their healthcare preferences and goals.

Policymakers and stakeholders are regularly consulted in order to determine the best ways to ensure there are incentives for engaging in AFHS. An essential component for driving change is consumer demand and educating the public about how they should insist on age-friendly environments and care settings. JAHF is also working in partnership with a variety of media organizations including WebMD and NBC to enhance public exposure to the resources available for older adults. To date, there are over 3000 care locations that have joined the age-friendly health systems movement and that number is growing nationally and internationally (Fulmer et al. 2020).

The USAging and its Aging and Disability Business Institute are focusing their efforts on collaborating with community-based organizations and healthcare systems to allow older adults with disabilities to gain easier access to necessary high-quality services and programs. They are specifically focusing on advancing integration, partnerships, and payment models between social services and health systems.

Case Study: The Age-Friendly Program in Portland.
In 2006 the city of Portland, through Portland State University's Institute on Aging, was the only city in the United States of America to participate in the original WHO Global Age-Friendly Cities project. The research for the project involved conducting a baseline assessment of the city's age friendliness. This gathered data through focus groups with older adults, caregivers of frail older people, and representatives of the public, business, and non-profit service sectors on age-friendly features and barriers in the city, as well as suggestions for improvements. Four years later, Portland (again through the university's Institute of Aging) became one of the original members of WHO's Global Network for Age-Friendly Cities and Communities. In 2013, the surrounding Multnomah County (one of 36 counties in the State of Oregon) was also accepted into the Network. The strength of Portland's age-friendly programme is its focus on making recommendations concerning City and County policies that, over the long run, will enhance the city's and county's age-friendliness. In some cases, the age-friendly coalition of stakeholders has reviewed and made recommendations for changes in policies, while other times it has suggested new policies (for example, equitable and affordable housing, transportation, employment practices). Currently, the city is attempting to expand age-friendly housing policies by focusing on local zoning codes revisions. The aim is to put accessible housing policy in place that requires and/or incentivizes accessible housing (no step entrances, wide halls and doors, and a bathroom and social space that can be visited by someone using a mobility device). Portland will continue to look for opportunities for involvement in projects and policies that will enhance age friendliness at the local level, from designing urban centres and transit corridors, to low-income utility programmes and the creation of accessible and affordable housing.

Source: Buffel et al. (n.d.)[1]

[1] This is an adaptation of an original work "Case Study: The Age-friendly Programme in Portland." Geneva: World Health Organization (WHO); n.d. Licence: CC BY-NC-SA 3.0 IGO. This adaptation was not created by WHO. WHO is not responsible for the content or accuracy of this adaptation. The original edition shall be the binding and authentic edition.

Acknowledgments The authors wish to gratefully acknowledge the editorial assistance of Abby Maglich, Intern, The John A. Hartford Foundation, Master of Healthcare Administration Candidate, Columbia University Mailman School of Public Health, in the preparation of this manuscript.

References

Ageing and Health. 2022. World Health Organization. https://www.who.int/news-room/fact-sheets/detail/ageing-and-health

Aung, M.N., Y. Koyanagi, S. Ueno, S. Tiraphat, and M. Yuasa. 2020. A Contemporary Insight into an Age-friendly Environment Contributing to the Social Network, Active Ageing and Quality of Life of Community Resident Seniors in Japan. *Journal of Aging and Environment* 35 (2): 145–160. https://doi.org/10.1080/26892618.2020.1813232.

Buffel, T., P. McGarry, C. Phillipson, L. De Donder, S. Dury, N. De Witte, A.S. Smetcoren, and D. Verté. 2014. Developing Age-friendly Cities: Case Studies From Brussels and Manchester and Implications for Policy and Practice. *Journal of Aging & Social Policy* 26 (1–2): 52–72. https://doi.org/10.1080/08959420.2014.855043.

Buffel, T., N. Cotterrell, C. Phillipson, S. Rémillard-Boilard, M. Neal, and A. D'eLa Torre. n.d. *Case Study: The Age-friendly Programme in Portland*. https://extranet.who.int/agefriendlyworld/resources/age-friendly-case-studies/portland/

Burke, R.E., L.E. Ashcraft, K. Manges, B. Kinosian, C.M. Lamberton, M.E. Bowen, R.T. Brown, S. Mavandadi, D.E. Hall, and R.M. Werner. 2022. What Matters When It Comes to Measuring Age-Friendly Health System Transformation. *Journal of the American Geriatrics Society* 70 (10): 2775–2785.

Busso, D.S., A. Volmert, and N. Kendall-Taylor. 2018. Reframing Aging: Effect of a Short-Term Framing Intervention on Implicit Measures of Age Bias. *The Journals of Gerontology: Series B* 74 (4): 559–564. https://doi.org/10.1093/geronb/gby080.

Butler, R.N. 1975. *Why Survive? Being Old in America*. Harper Torchbooks.

Chao, T.S., and H. Huang. 2016. The East Asian Age-friendly Cities Promotion – Taiwan's Experience and the Need for an Oriental Paradigm. *Global Health Promotion* 23 (1 Suppl): 85–89. https://doi.org/10.1177/1757975916641612.

Chatters, L.M., H.O. Taylor, and R.J. Taylor. 2020. Older Black Americans During COVID-19: Race and Age Double Jeopardy. *Health Education & Behavior* 47 (6): 855–860. https://doi.org/10.1177/1090198120965513.

Dash, K., J. Shue, T. Driver, A. Bonner, L. Pelton, R. Snyder, A. Diep, S. Espinosa, and T. Fulmer. 2022. Developing a Shared Language to Describe the Age-Friendly Ecosystem: Technical Meeting Report. *International Journal of Geriatrics and Gerontology* 6 (1): 10.29011/2577-0748.100034.

De Biasi, A., M. Wolfe, J. Carmody, T. Fulmer, and J. Auerbach. 2020. Creating an Age-Friendly Public Health System. *Innovation in Aging* 4 (1): 1–11. https://doi.org/10.1093/geroni/igz044.

Du, Y., and Q. Xu. 2016. Health Disparities and Delayed Health Care among Older Adults in California: A Perspective from Race, Ethnicity, and Immigration. *Public Health Nursing* 33 (5): 383–394. https://doi.org/10.1111/phn.12260.

Durant, T.J., Jr. 2011. The Utility of Vulnerability and Social Capital Theories in Studying the Impact of Hurricane Katrina on the Elderly. *Journal of Family Issues* 32 (10): 1285–1302.

Fitzgerald, K.G., and F.G. Caro. 2014. An Overview of Age-Friendly Cities and Communities Around the World. *Journal of Aging & Social Policy* 26 (1–2): 1–18. https://doi.org/10.1080/08959420.2014.860786.

Fulmer, T., A. Berman, K. Mate, and L. Pelton. 2020. Age-Friendly Health Systems: The 4Ms. *Best Pract Nurs Care Older Adults* 35: 1–2.

Hayes-Larson, E., T.M. Mobley, A. Gilmore-Bykovskyi, C. Shaw, A. Karlamangla, J.J. Manly, and E.R. Mayeda. 2021. Racial/Ethnic Differences in Health-Related Quality of Life in Persons With and Without Dementia. *Journal of the American Geriatrics Society* 69 (3): 629–636.

Hung, L., A. Hudson, M. Gregorio, L. Jackson, J. Mann, N. Horne, A. Berndt, C. Wallsworth, L. Wong, and A. Phinney. 2021. Creating Dementia-Friendly Communities for Social Inclusion: A Scoping Review. *Gerontology and Geriatric Medicine* 7: 23337214211013596. https://doi.org/10.1177/23337214211013596.

Jacobson, G., Cicchiello, A., Shah, A., M.M. Doty, and R.D. Williams. 2021. *When Costs Are a Barrier To Getting Health Care: Reports from Older Adults in the United States and Other High-Income Countries* (Commonwealth Fund, Oct. 2021).

Kalache, A., I. Hoskins, and S. Mende. 2004. *Towards Age-friendly Primary Health Care*. http://www.emro.who.int/images/stories/elderly/documents/Towards_Age_Freindly_PHC.pdf?ua=1

Kim, K., T.D. Buckley, D. Burnette, J. Huang, and S. Kim. 2022. Age-friendly Communities and Older Adults' Health in the United States. *International Journal of Environmental Research and Public Health* 19 (15). https://doi.org/10.3390/ijerph19159292.

Korte, M., J. Graupner, K. Thompson, and L.J. Gleason. 2022. Age Friendly Care: What Do Community Aging Services Professionals Need to Know? *Gerontology & Geriatrics Education* 28: 1–10. https://doi.org/10.1080/02701960.2022.2151443.

Landefeld, C.S., R.M. Palmer, D.M. Kresevic, R.H. Fortinsky, and J. Kowal. 1995. A Randomized Trial of Care in a Hospital Medical Unit Especially Designed to Improve the Functional Outcomes of Acutely Ill Older Patients. *New England Journal of Medicine* 332 (20): 1338–1344.

Langley, G.J., R.D. Moen, K.M. Nolan, T.W. Nolan, C.L. Norman, and L.P. Provost. 2009. *The Improvement Guide: A Practical Approach to Enhancing Organizational Performance*. Wiley.

Levy, S.R. 2018. Toward Reducing Ageism: PEACE (Positive Education About Aging and Contact Experiences) Model. *The Gerontologist* 58 (2): 226–232. https://doi.org/10.1093/geront/gnw116.

Mate, K., T. Fulmer, L. Pelton, A. Berman, A. Bonner, W. Huang, and J. Zhang. 2021. Evidence for the 4Ms: Interactions and Outcomes Across the Care Continuum. *Journal of Aging and Health* 33 (7–8): 469–481. https://doi.org/10.1177/0898264321991658.

Montepare, J.M., and L.M. Brown. 2022. Age-friendly Universities (AFU): Combating and Inoculating Against Ageism in a Pandemic and Beyond. *Journal of Social Issues* 78 (4): 1017–1037. https://doi.org/10.1111/josi.12541.

Ouslander, J.G., and D.C. Grabowski. 2020. COVID-19 in Nursing Homes: Calming the Perfect Storm. *Journal of the American Geriatrics Society* 68 (10): 2153–2162.

Reuben, D.B., L.C. Evertson, R. Jackson-Stoeckle, G. Epstein-Lubow, L.H. Spragens, K.L. Haggerty, K.S. Serrano, and L.A. Jennings. 2022. Dissemination of a Successful Dementia Care Program: Lessons to Facilitate Spread of Innovations. *Journal of the American Geriatrics Society* 70 (9): 2686–2694. https://doi.org/10.1111/jgs.17900.

Rhee, T.G., R.A. Marottoli, P.H. Van Ness, and B.R. Levy. 2019. Impact of Perceived Racism on Healthcare Access Among Older Minority Adults. *American Journal of Preventive Medicine* 56 (4): 580–585. https://doi.org/10.1016/j.amepre.2018.10.010.

The John A. Hartford Foundation. n.d.. The *Age-friendly Ecosystem: Sectors and Initiatives [Infographic]*. Retrieved from https://www.johnahartford.org/grants-strategy/current-strategies/age-friendly/age-friendly-ecosystem

Wolfe, M., and J.N. Gracia. 2023. The Value of Age-Friendly Public Health Systems in the Age-friendly Ecosystem. *Geriatrics* 8 (3): 63. https://doi.org/10.3390/geriatrics8030063.

Chapter 2
Age-Friendliness as a Framework for Equity in Aging

Valerie Chang Greer and Linda S. Edelman

Health exists inside social and environmental contexts. Consider the following vignettes. A 76-year-old immigrant moves to live with her daughter after falling and breaking her hip. A 78-year-old African American man contracts COVID from his teenage grandson and spends 14 days alone in his apartment until he tests negative. A 90-year-old White woman living alone in her suburban home suddenly experiences shortness of breath and tingling in her legs and calls 911. A retired Indigenous couple, both 75-years old and beginning to show declines in memory, move across the country to live in a retirement community near their children and grandchildren, leaving behind their ancestral homeland. The events preceding and following these snapshots are nuanced—influenced by past environments, and Social Determinants of Health (SDOH), which impact what follows. SDOH are distal upstream drivers of health and are major predictors of how an individual will age. Concurrently, the factor of place plays an active, vital role in SDOH and health and well-being, and the qualities of places are known to have a particularly significant impact on people in later years of life.

V. C. Greer (✉)
College of Architecture and Planning, School of Architecture, Healthy Aging and Resilient Places Lab, The University of Utah, Salt Lake City, UT, USA
e-mail: valerie.greer@utah.edu

L. S. Edelman
College of Nursing, Hartford Center of Geriatric Nursing Excellence, Utah Geriatric Education Consortium (UGEC), Utah Rural Opioid Consortium Collaborative Care Model (UROHC-CCM), The University of Utah, Salt Lake City, UT, USA

V. Chang Greer, L. S. Edelman (eds.), *Age-Friendly Ecosystems*, SpringerBriefs in Public Health, https://doi.org/10.1007/978-3-031-68361-9_2

Introduction

Inequities in aging and the prominence of place are well documented (Barrett 2022; O'rand 2018; Silva et al. 2019). The "zip code paradigm" recognizes that a zip code is a stronger determinant of health and life expectancy than a genetic code (Graham et al. 2015). Life expectancy can vary by 20–30 years among people living just a few miles away from each other, and up to as much as 41 years among census tracks in the United States (Neuroscience News 2018). Research shows as much as 60 percent of health may be attributed to the zip code where one resides (Morgan 2019). Current models can predict differences in life expectancy even within zip codes, based on census track-level data (Robert Wood Johnson Foundation n.d.). This underscores the interrelationship between place and health and points to disparate conditions in physical environments that shape experiences of aging.

The SDOH that make zip codes strong determinants of health are complex and include income, education, environmental factors, crime, and access to food, housing, and health care, to name a few. Health inequities arise from the overlapping relationships among SDOH and race and, when considering older adults, ageism. The World Health Organization recognizes that SDOH are responsible in large part for health inequities between and within countries in the statement: "This unequal distribution of health-damaging experiences is not in any sense a 'natural' phenomenon but is a result of a toxic combination of poor social policies and programmes, unfair economic arrangements, and bad politics" (WHO Commission on Social Determinants of Health, & World Health Organization 2008). Place-based disparities that impact aging are also not "natural." The late leader in minority aging research, Steven Wallace, argues that the greatest challenges of growing old may not be medical but rather social and political processes, as evidenced by the inequities among older adults based on race, gender, class, and citizenship status (Wallace 2021).

Structural racism contributes to stark inequities in aging through social, economic, and environmental mechanisms (Garcia et al. 2021; Gee and Ford 2011; Sewell 2016). People in racial and ethnic minority groups are more likely to experience illness and death across a wide range of chronic health conditions, including diabetes, hypertension, obesity, asthma, and heart disease, when compared to their White counterparts (Centers for Disease Control and Prevention 2021). Deeply rooted inequalities in economic stability, housing security, and investment in health and education accumulate across domains, generations, and the life course, contributing to weathering processes and age patterns of allostatic load, characterized greater physiological dysregulation, inflammation, and accelerated biological aging among adults in minoritized populations (Crimmins and Seeman 2004; Garcia et al. 2021; Geronimus et al. 2006; Goosby et al. 2018). Negative health effects stemming from structural racism seen through aging populations must be recognized in relationship to a web of physical and social environments, and within a much larger life-course perspective.

Health disparities from COVID-19 have magnified the uneven distribution of resources among communities and highlighted the vulnerability this creates for people in racial and ethnic minority populations (Willems et al. 2022). Spatial models of COVID testing results show that demographic, socioeconomic, and racial characteristics play an important role in higher positive testing rates (DiMaggio et al. 2020). Built-environment level factors that are seen to be drivers of disease include population density and housing density (CDC Covid-19 Response Team 2020; Florida 2020). Age-adjusted data show that people of color are disproportionately impacted by COVID-19, and that Black people are about twice as likely to die from COVID-19 as their White counterparts (Hill and Artiga 2022). Over 80 percent of total COVID-19 deaths for the first 2 years of the pandemic were among older adults (CDC Covid-19 Response Team 2020), and this proportion increased to almost 90 percent by the end of 2022 (Haanschoten et al. 2023). Not only were older adults more likely to die from COVID-19, but they also experienced high levels of social isolation and loneliness, depression, and reduced quality of life (Kasar and Karaman 2021). Disparities within the United States among older adults and people in racial and ethnic minority populations are witnessed in other parts of the world. This sobering view of inequity stemming from COVID-19 demonstrates how deep disparities run in the social, economic, and environmental places we live.

This chapter examines the origins, development, and future of the age-friendly movement as a critical framework for recognizing social and environmental factors that shape aging. We argue that the lens of equity must widen significantly in future discourse and that the ambition of age-friendly agendas should extend to focus on addressing social, environmental, and health disparities. The age-friendly movement has a unique capacity to be influential, having been established with both a "ground up" and "top-down" approach to aging services, health care, research, and collaboration. Local-level initiatives are imperative to understanding unique physical and social constructs distinct to cultures and geographies. At the same time, state and national public policy and action are critical to addressing historic patterns of marginalization, underrepresentation, and discrimination and to tackling larger global challenges such as climate change and urban migration as they impact aging populations. The capacity of the age-friendly movement to work both locally and globally makes it a driver in reconceptualizing knowledge about the heterogeneity of older adult populations and centering the voices of older adults themselves, particularly those who have historically been subordinated by systems of power. Considering how the age-friendly movement has grown to impact design and placemaking in a variety of settings, we identify the value of an intersectional approach to future age-friendly work to reflect the diversity within older adult populations. The age-friendly movement has tremendous potential to drive much-needed change, yet to create truly impactful age-friendly ecosystems, the need for equity in aging must be addressed in new ways.

Origins of the Age-Friendly Movement

The need to address rapid population aging and the accompanying social transformation was first recognized on a global stage by the UN Assembly General in 1978. The First World Assembly on Aging was convened in 1982, and the International Plan of Action on Aging was adopted in Vienna as the first international instrument on aging (United Nations 1982); this plan includes 62 recommendations that range from research, training, and education to improvements in health and nutrition, the built environment, and social welfare. In order to bring international attention to issues of aging and support countries and states in addressing the needs of growing populations of older adults, the UN designated an International Day of Older Persons in 1991 and proclaimed 1999 as the International Year of Older Persons (United Nations 1999). These designations were significant in putting aging and research onto international political agendas, calling government decision-makers, researchers, practitioners, community associations, and the public at large to focus on developments in aging (Andrews and Clark 1999).

The paradigm of "active aging" was central to early conceptualizations of age-friendly cities and communities, which emerged in the early 2000s (Buffel et al. 2018). Active aging was defined by the World Health Organization (WHO) in 2002 as the ability for people to participate in social, cultural, civic, spiritual, and economic matters in old age (World Health Organization n.d.). The WHO called for active aging policies and programs to improve both social and physical environments. Also in 2002, the Second World Assembly on Ageing was convened, and the Madrid International Plan of Action on Ageing was adopted to respond to challenges and opportunities of population aging. The Plan of Action recognizes that the global demographic shift in aging is resulting in "Profound consequences for every aspect of individual, community, national, and international life" and identifies three priority directions: advancing health, ensuring supportive environments, and promoting participation in development (United Nations 2002).

This work set the stage for the launch of the WHO "Global Age-friendly Cities" project in 2006. The project hosted a series of focus groups with older people, caregivers, and service providers in 33 cities and 22 countries in order to identify factors that make urban environments more "age-friendly." Data from these international focus groups resulted in the publication of the WHO's *Global Age-friendly Cities: A Guide*, which examines characteristics of an age-friendly city (AFC) in three main areas: service provision, social aspects, and the built environment (World Health Organization 2007). The Age-friendly Cities framework identifies eight interconnected domains which help identify and address barriers to the well-being and participation of older people, including (1) safe and reliable transportation; (2) housing options and services that support older adults aging in place; (3) accessible and safe outdoor spaces, including parks and buildings; (4) opportunities for older adults to remain engaged in learning, cultural, and social activities; (5) respect for the wisdom of older adults and social inclusion of all ages and cultures; (6) civic participation and employment opportunities that encourage older adults to utilize their skills to strengthen communities; (7) accessible and affordable health services; and 8) communication structures that provide information and technology allowing older adults to take advantage of community resources and services (World Health Organization n.d.).

Thus, the birth of the age-friendly movement linked twin challenges of population aging and rapid urbanization and recognized the role of environment in healthy aging (Noordzij et al. 2019). From its inception, the age-friendly movement has strongly emphasized participation and contributions from older adults, recognizing the differences between communities and political institutions and reflecting a vision of a "bottom-up" or grassroots promotion of age-friendly communities in parallel with global support for aging (Fitzgerald and Caro 2014). This work stems from community coproduction and is significant because partnerships and practices that are possible in one location are not necessarily transferable to another. Places themselves represent a wide spectrum of ages—for instance, there are young and old cities; the pace of aging within places also ranges—for instance, from "fast aging" to "slow aging" of populations (van Hoof et al. 2021). As such, the study of age-friendly places must be understood as a highly dynamic and changing condition that is characterized by its unique relationship with the evolving nature of place.

Early manifestations of age-friendly practices in the United States were seen with the formation of the Certified Age-Friendly Employer (CAFE) initiative in 2006, which promoted workplaces free of age discrimination; multi-sectoral initiatives began in tandem, such as Age-Friendly New York City, which was formed in 2007 as a collaboration between the Office of the Mayor, the New York City Council, and the New York Academy of Medicine. The notion of "lifetime" neighborhoods in the United Kingdom and naturally occurring retirement communities (NORC) in the United States gained attention in public and planning discourse in 2008 and 2009 (Buffel et al. 2012). Multiple models of age-friendly housing have since emerged internationally and can be understood within three broad categories: age-adapted homes in mainstream housing, specialized, alternative models such as cohousing and retirement villages, and congregate care settings (van Hoof et al. 2021). In 2010, the WHO launched the Global Network for age-friendly cities and communities (AFCC), an online portal for the exchange of knowledge and data on age-friendly initiatives that promote cross-nation dialogue. The network currently represents 1445 cities in 51 countries and plays an important role in promoting knowledge exchange about age-friendly places across a global scale.

In tandem with the emergence of the AFCC Global Network, there has been a proliferation of ways that age-friendliness has extended to place types and settings. In 2012, Dublin City University developed the Ten Principles of Age-friendly Universities and formally launched the Age-Friendly University (AFU) Global Network, which advances age inclusivity within educational opportunities, research agendas, community engagement, and access to resources and activities. As of the time of this writing, there are over 50 colleges and universities that have received age-friendly designation, representing schools in the United States, Europe, Canada, and Asia. Adoption of AFU principles varies among institutions, yet three themes emerge as common threads: interdisciplinary collaboration within the university, partnerships with community, and alignment with global priorities and initiatives (Montepare and Brown 2022).

The Age-Friendly Health Systems Initiative was launched in 2016 by the John A. Hartford Foundation and the Institute of Healthcare Improvement (IHI) in partnership with the American Hospital Association (AHA) and the Catholic Health Association of the United States (CHA). The conceptual framework guiding age-friendly health systems is known as the 4Ms: What Matters, Medication, Mentation, and Mobility (Fulmer et al. 2020). As of the time of this writing, over 3000 healthcare sites in the United States are part of the Age-Friendly Health Systems movement. Shared among these initiatives is the premise that a range of interventions are required to support healthy aging, and that the multidisciplinary work needed to create age-friendly environments can be promoted and advanced through common aims and principles. This broad conceptualization of the collaboration required between environments and disciplines to support health sets the foundation for creating age-friendly ecosystems (Fulmer et al. 2020).

Thus, in a relatively short period of time, age-friendliness has grown from the context of cities into domains of neighborhoods, universities, public health, and health systems. Globally, there is a spectrum of scales by which age-friendly initiatives receive funding and operate. For instance, Age-Friendly Environments in Europe (AFEE) represents a multinational commitment to bring together a collection of lessons learned from large and small age-friendly cities and communities throughout the European Union. Taiwan and Singapore, which are expected to be classified as superaged societies by 2026, have consistently received strong governmental support to advance age-friendly environments. In the United States, there are over 500 communities that participate in the AARP Network of Age-Friendly Cities and Communities; participants in this age-friendly network commit to a 5-year process that includes a community assessment, the development of a comprehensive plan and a period of implementation (Dabelko-Schoeny and White 2021). While age-friendliness has made a significant impact in wealthy developed countries, factors in developing nations such as poor economic conditions, unavailability of information about the needs of aging populations, or lack of governmental support may make support for age-friendly initiatives seem out of reach, (Fitzgerald and Caro 2014). There is a need for longitudinal and cross-national studies that account for the temporal characteristics of place and recognize that contemporary patterns of urban development reflect huge variations (Noordzij et al. 2019; Woolrych et al. 2022).

Contemporary Criticism: Age-Friendly for Whom?

Criticism of the age-friendly movement calls attention to a need for greater inclusion and the ability to address diversity among older adult populations (Buffel et al. 2018; Handler 2018; Meeks 2022). Within the domain of cities, the AFC agenda has been criticized for lacking relevance to developing regions and low-income settings, leading to a call for the future development of an "age-friendly slums" initiative (Aboderin et al. 2017). Questions have been raised about whether design principles, which are often derived from problem-solving and summarized into recommendations, can adequately account for the diversity of local contexts and heterogeneity of older adult populations (Buffel et al. 2012; Handler 2018). Multiple aspects of diversity, ranging from neurodiversity to ethnic and socioeconomic diversity, point to different characteristics that become particularly important within the context of cities; for instance, in asking how "age-friendly" might be experienced by an older adult with vision impairment, Peace et al. (2018) found that technology adoption of cities, street and sidewalk design, and transportation were specifically important to promote a sense of social inclusion among visually impaired older adult residents. In addition, AFC work has been criticized for standing apart from larger, global urban policies and movements, such as urban migration and climate change (Noordzij et al. 2019). To date, there has been limited exchange between the AFC movement and discourse in urban geography, planning, and design around significant changes in metropolitan areas, including widening socioeconomic inequalities, privatization of public space, and rise of global cities (Handler 2018; Noordzij et al. 2019). These global trends, which often result in the displacement of older adults from urban cores, fundamentally challenge the concept of an age-friendly city and require greater study and response.

Criticism of the age-friendly university movement largely centers around concerns over equity in the twin realms of education and research. Barriers that may hinder older adults from participating in higher education are known, but less is known about how to address those barriers (Hansen et al. 2019). Research is needed to understand course design strategies, classroom dynamics, and age-related differences among students who contribute to productive intergenerational exchange (Montepare and Brown 2022). There is also a need to address systemic-level challenges related to expanding age diversity on campuses, including acclimation, stressors, career concerns, return on investment, and ageism (Morrow-Howell et al. 2020). In the realm of research, the field of aging studies has historically been criticized for being focused on predominantly White, English-speaking, and resourced populations (Chinn et al. 2021). The underrepresentation of minoritized and underserved populations in aging research reflects a need to address established barriers including transportation, language, financial, and logistical challenges (Gilmore-Bykovskyi et al. 2022). There is a need for more cross-cultural and cross-country comparisons in aging research to better understand how theoretical approaches to policies and programs vary within different physical, socioeconomic, and cultural contexts (Blessett et al. 2019). There is also a need for longitudinal and cross-national studies that account for the temporal characteristics of place (Noordzij et al. 2019; Woolrych et al. 2022).

Critical themes resonate within the age-friendly health movement. The traditional focus on clinical relationships and technologies in the field of bioethics has resulted in unresolved questions about the broader distribution of health and the institutional contexts within which clinical relationships operate (Daniels 2006). It is known that differential exposures to stressful environments serve as a major factor in widening health disparities as we age, yet there is a knowledge gap in how structural inequities in the places we live contribute to major health disparities and outcomes (Chinn et al. 2021). Additionally, there has been increased international attention to ageism as a pernicious detriment to physical and mental health (Chang et al. 2020) and a critical reflection on human rights in older age (Hopf et al. 2020). Socio-scientific and political debate on age discrimination has resonated around the justification of "age limits" and age-based prioritization of health resources, such as seen in the COVID-19 response (Farrell et al. 2020). Further, older adults living in nursing homes experienced high mortality rates from COVID-19, particularly for racial and ethnic minorities on Medicaid (Gorges and Konetzka 2021). These differences illuminated by the disparities in care that vulnerable older adults dependent on long-term services and supports experience (Rivera-Hernandez et al. 2019; Shippee et al. 2022).

Collectively, criticism of age-friendliness in the contexts of cities, campuses, and health systems calls attention to the need to broaden the reach of those *who* participate in age-friendly places. While the age-friendly movement has made significant global contributions in conceptualizing frameworks for improving access, mobility, services, and safety and in creating a framework for multi-sectoral collaboration, there is an urgent call to account for the complex webs of challenges that present barriers to aging well, particularly for marginalized and underserved populations. Interactions and relationships with environments are fundamentally shaped by differences among people, including cognitive and physical abilities, socioeconomic advantage/disadvantage, ethnicity, and personal historical influences such as trauma (Meeks 2022). Contemporary discourse and future trajectories need to address social inequalities, health disparities, and exclusion as a central focus of age-friendly scholarship and initiatives in order to advance equity in aging (Buffel et al. 2018).

An Intersectional Approach to Addressing Inequities in Aging

Future directions in the age-friendly movement may benefit from an intersectional approach to the complexities that link social and physical environments with identities and experiences (Wilkinson et al. 2023). The concept of intersectionality (Crenshaw 1989) highlights how multiple social forces and identities, including gender, race, sexuality, and ethnicity, do not operate as individual or exclusive entities, but rather as reciprocally constructing phenomena. By adopting an intersectional lens, emerging age-friendly work might recognize that "focus on the most privileged group members marginalizes those who are multiply burdened and obscures claims that cannot be understood as resulting from discrete sources of discrimination" (Crenshaw 1989). This concept harbors significance to future age-friendly work as ageism is widely recognized as a deeply rooted, and even socially acceptable form, of bias (American Psychological Association 2023). The stereotypes that abound within public attitudes toward aging belie the diversity of experiences that converge within aging populations, and the myriad ways that age-friendly environments play influential roles to shape meaningful engagement. In response to age-related stereotypes and biases, the concept of intersectionality begins to advance a more productive public narrative about aging by focusing on the overlaps of social forces and identities and resisting over-simplistic classifications.

As an analytic tool, intersectionality has the potential to advance age-friendly work by describing how different forms of bias are linked with institutional organizations of power, such as those that shape place-based domains of housing, education, and health.

> Intersectionality is a way of understanding and analyzing the complexity in the world, in people, and in human experiences…When it comes to social inequity, people's lives and the organization of power in a given society are better understood as being shaped not by a single axis of social division, be it race or gender or class, but by many axes that work together and influence each other. Intersectionality as an analytic tool gives people better access to the complexity of the world and of themselves. (Bilge and Hill Collins 2016)

This analytical approach aligns with the groundwork established within the age-friendly movement that emphasizes the relationality and the plurality of experiences people have with the places they live. There is a need to understand power structures that shape placemaking through intersectional lenses, and as pathways that contribute to persistent, structural inequities. Intersectionality as an analytical tool also underscores the significance of coproducing knowledge that is specific to locations, cultures, and communities; furthermore, by bringing social contexts into consideration, intersectional approaches insist upon a way of understanding social inequity in relational terms. This form of analysis creates a framework for the devolution of "us" vs "them," or the "othering" of older adult populations while also calling attention to the active role that organizations of power play in constructing dynamics of equity.

Beyond the conceptualization and use of intersectionality as an analytical tool, intersectionality has been influential in policy and attempts to tackle health-related outcomes. Intersectionality is understood as more than a sum of parts, and so too must social, economic, and environmental power structures be considered as a calculus of factors that contribute to aging across the lifespan. This is particularly true regarding health equities. The 4 M framework guiding age-friendly health systems guides holistic health care that honors what matters most to older adults and their caregivers. However, it is impossible to honor the care preferences without considering the social and cultural milieu that comprises the older adult's physical and emotional environments. Increasingly, the intersections of old age, environmental conditions, and social categories guide an understanding of vulnerabilities that lead to health disparities, which in turn inform policy recommendations (Conteh et al. 2021). It is fundamentally important to consider the plethora of social axes that combine with physical environments and personal identities to create health outcomes over the life-course.

Conclusion: A Case of Need for Equity in Aging

Age-friendliness has proliferated from a response to rapid urbanization and demographic change into a social movement. The work of today focuses on connecting places to generate larger age-friendly ecosystems. This requires new forms of collaboration and design thinking that fundamentally consider the case of the need for equity in aging. As the global demographic transforms and the population of older adults becomes the most heterogeneous of all ages, the time is ripe to take a critical look at the conception of equity within age-friendly initiatives: age-friendly for whom; age-friendly where; and how can age-friendly places address the complex social, economic, and physical barriers that contribute to massive disparities within aging populations? The following chapters in this book consider initiatives and ideas within the domains of age-friendly neighborhoods, campuses, and health systems, which were the focus of the Age-friendly Communities Symposium in 2022. Perspectives from a World Café hosted for participants of the symposium are highlighted in order to consider the intersection of these domains in the Intermountain West region of the United States. Authors examine the capacity for transformative work within each place-based domain that broadens the reach of who is reached in age-friendly environments and connects to a larger conception of age-friendly ecosystems. Equally as important, authors consider how the synergies between place-based settings intersect and support each other in efforts to radically reshape inclusivity in aging.

References

Aboderin, I., M. Kano, and H.A. Owii. 2017. Toward 'Age-Friendly Slums'? Health Challenges of Older Slum Dwellers in Nairobi and the Applicability of the Age-Friendly City Approach. *International Journal of Environmental Research and Public Health* 14 (10): 1259.

American Psychological Association. 2023. https://www.apa.org/monitor/2023/03/cover-new-concept-of-aging

Andrews, G., and M.J. Clark. 1999. The International Year of Older Persons: Putting Aging and Research Onto the Political Agenda. *The Journals of Gerontology Series B: Psychological Sciences and Social Sciences* 54 (1): P7–P10.

Barrett, A.E. 2022. Centering Age Inequality: Developing a Sociology-of-Age Framework. *Annual Review of Sociology* 48: 213–232.

Bilge, S., and P.H. Collins. 2016. *Intersectionality*. Cambridge: Polity.

Blessett, Brandi, Jennifer Dodge, Beverly Edmond, Holly T. Goerdel, Susan T. Gooden, Andrea M. Headley, Norma M. Riccucci, and Brian N. Williams. 2019. Social Equity in Public Administration: A Call to Action. *Perspectives on Public Management and Governance* 2 (4): 283–299.

Buffel, T., C. Phillipson, and T. Scharf. 2012. Ageing in Urban Environments: Developing 'Age-Friendly Cities. *Critical Social Policy* 32 (4): 597–617.

Buffel, T., S. Handler, and C. Phillipson. 2018. *Age-Friendly Cities and Communities*. Bristol: Policy Press.

CDC Covid-19 Response Team. 2020. Geographic Differences in COVID-19 Cases, Deaths, and Incidence – United States, February 12–April 7, 2020. *Morbidity and Mortality Weekly Report* 69 (15): 465–471.

Centers for Disease Control and Prevention. 2021. *Racism and Health*. Centers for Disease Control and Prevention. Retrieved March 21, 2023, from https://www.cdc.gov/minorityhealth/racism-disparities/index.html

Chang, E-Shien, Sneha Kannoth, Samantha Levy, Shi-Yi Wang, John E. Lee, and Becca R. Levy. 2020. Global Reach of Ageism on Older Persons' Health: A Systematic Review. *PLoS One* 15 (1): e0220857.

Chinn, J.J., I.K. Martin, and N. Redmond. 2021. Health Equity Among Black Women in the United States. *Journal of Women's Health* 30 (2): 212–219.

Conteh, A., A. Wilkinson, and J. Macarthy. 2021. Exploring Gender, Health, and Intersectionality in Informal Settlements in Freetown. *Gender and Development* 29 (1): 111–129.

Crenshaw, K. 1989. Demarginalizing the Intersection of Race and Sex: A Black Feminist Critique of Antidiscrimination Doctrine, Feminist Theory and Antiracist Politics. *University of Chicago Legal Forum*: Vol. 1989, Article 8. Available at https://chicagounbound.uchicago.edu/uclf/vol1989/iss1/8

Crimmins, E.M., and T.E. Seeman. 2004. Integrating Biology into the Study of Health Disparities. *Population and Development Review* 30: 89–107.

Dabelko-Schoeny, H., and K. White. 2021. *What It Takes to Be and Remain an Age-Friendly World*. Generations. Retrieved November 23, 2023, from https://generations.asaging.org/how-be-and-remain-age-friendly-world

Daniels, N. 2006. Equity and Population Health: Toward a Broader Bioethics Agenda. *The Hastings Center Report* 36 (4): 22–35.

DiMaggio, C., M. Klein, C. Berry, and S. Frangos. 2020. Black/African American Communities Are at Highest Risk of COVID-19: Spatial Modeling of New York City ZIP Code–level Testing Results. *Annals of Epidemiology* 51: 7–13.

Farrell, Timothy W., Lauren E. Ferrante, Teneille Brown, Leslie Francis, Eric Widera, Ramona Rhodes, Tony Rosen, et al. 2020. AGS Position Statement: Resource Allocation Strategies and Age-related Considerations in the COVID-19 Era and Beyond. *Journal of the American Geriatrics Society* 68 (6): 1136–1142.

Fitzgerald, K.G., and F.G. Caro. 2014. An Overview of Age-Friendly Cities and Communities Around the World. *Journal of Aging & Social Policy* 26 (1–2): 1–18. https://doi.org/10.1080/08959420.2014.860786.

Florida, R. 2020. *The Geography of Coronavirus*. Bloomberg CITYLAB. https://www.bloomberg.com/news/articles/2020-04-03/what-we-know-about-density-and-covid-19-s-spread

Fulmer, T., P. Patel, N. Levy, K. Mate, A. Berman, L. Pelton, J. Beard, A. Kalache, and J. Auerbach. 2020. Moving Toward a Global Age-Friendly Ecosystem. *Journal of the American Geriatrics Society* 68 (9): 1936–1940. https://doi.org/10.1111/jgs.16675.

Garcia, M.A., P.A. Homan, C. García, and T.H. Brown. 2021. The Color of COVID-19: Structural Racism and the Disproportionate Impact of the Pandemic on Older Black and Latinx Adults. *The Journals of Gerontology: Series B* 76 (3): e75–e80. https://doi.org/10.1093/geronb/gbaa114.

Gee, G.C., and C.L. Ford. 2011. Structural Racism and Health Inequities: Old issues, New Directions. *Du Bois Review: Social Science Research on Race* 8 (1): 115–132.

Geronimus, A.T., M. Hicken, D. Keene, and J. Bound. 2006. 'Weathering' and Age Patterns of Allostatic Load Scores Among Blacks and Whites in the United States. *American Journal of Public Health* 96 (5): 826–833.

Gilmore-Bykovskyi, A., R. Croff, C.M. Glover, J.D. Jackson, J. Resendez, A. Perez, M. Zuelsdorff, G. Green-Harris, and J.J. Manly. 2022. Traversing the Aging Research and Health Equity Divide: Toward Intersectional Frameworks of Research Justice and Participation. *The Gerontologist* 62 (5): 711–720.

Goosby, B.J., J.E. Cheadle, and C. Mitchell. 2018. Stress-related Biosocial Mechanisms of Discrimination and African American Health Inequities. *Annual Review of Sociology* 44: 319–340. https://doi.org/10.1146/annurev-soc-060116-053403.

Gorges, R.J., and R.T. Konetzka. 2021. Factors Associated with Racial Differences in Deaths Among Nursing Home Residents With COVID-19 Infection in the US. *JAMA Network Open* 4 (2): e2037431.

Graham, G., M.L. Ostrowski, and A. Sabrina. 2015. *Defeating the ZIP Code Health Paradigm: Data, Technology, And Collaboration Are Key. HealthAffairs*. Retrieved March 22, 2023, from https://www.healthaffairs.org/do/10.1377/forefront.20150806.049730

Haanschoten, E., H. Dubendris, H.E. Reses, et al. 2023. Disparities in COVID-19 Vaccination Status Among Long-Term Care Facility Residents – United States, October 31, 2022–May 7, 2023. *Morbitity and Mortality Weekly Report* 72: 1095–1098. https://doi.org/10.15585/mmwr.mm7240a4.

Handler, S. 2018. Alternative Age-Friendly Initiatives: Redefining Age-Friendly Design. In *Age-Friendly Cities and Communities*, 211–230. Policy Press.

Hansen, R.J., C.A. Talmage, S.P. Thaxton, and R.C. Knopf. 2019. Barriers to Age-Friendly Universities (AFU): Lessons from Osher Lifelong Learning Institute Demographics and Perceptions. *Gerontology & Geriatrics Education* 40 (2): 221–243. https://doi.org/10.1080/02701960.2019.1572003.

Hill, L., and S. Artiga. 2022. *Covid-19 Cases and Deaths by Race/ethnicity: Current Data and Changes Over Time*. KFF. Retrieved March 21, 2023, from https://www.kff.org/coronavirus-covid-19/issue-brief/covid-19-cases-and-deaths-by-race-ethnicity-current-data-and-changes-over-time/

Hopf, S., F. Previtali, and N. Georgantzi. 2020. Human Rights in Older Age: A Critical Reflection of the Debate Around a UN Convention on the Rights of Older Persons. *Innovation in Aging* 4 (Suppl 1): 19–20.

Kasar, K.S., and E. Karaman. 2021. Life in Lockdown: Social Isolation, Loneliness and Quality of Life in the Elderly During the COVID-19 Pandemic: A Scoping Review. *Geriatric Nursing* 42 (5): 1222–1229. https://doi.org/10.1016/j.gerinurse.2021.03.010.

Meeks, S. 2022. Age-Friendly Communities: Introduction to the Special Issue. *The Gerontologist* 62 (1): 1–5.

Montepare, J.M., and L.M. Brown. 2022. Age-Friendly Universities (AFU): Combating and Inoculating Against Ageism in a Pandemic and Beyond. *Journal of Social Issues* 78 (3): 1017–1037.

Morgan, K. 2019. *Story from Blue Cross Blue Shield Association: Up to 60% of Our Health is Determined by ZIP Code*. USA Today. Retrieved March 21, 2023, from https://www.usatoday.com/story/sponsor-story/blue-cross-blue-shield-association/2019/04/22/up-60-our-health-determined-zip-code/3542001002/

Morrow-Howell, N., N. Galucia, E. Swinford, and T. Meyer. 2020. Challenges and Opportunities of Age Diverse Universities: Perspectives from Admissions and Career Services. *Gerontology & Geriatrics Education* 43 (3): 328–345.

Neuroscience News. 2018. *Being Born in the Wrong Zip Code Can Shorten Your Life*. Neuroscience News. Retrieved March 21, 2023, from https://neurosciencenews.com/life-expectancy-zip-code-10018/

Noordzij, J.M., M.A. Beenackers, A.V.D. Roux, and F.J. van Lenthe. 2019. Age-Friendly Cities: Challenges for Future Research. *Bulletin of the World Health Organization* 97 (6): 436–437.

O'rand, A. 2018. *Age and Inequality: Diverse Pathways Through Later Life*. Routledge.

Peace, S., J. Katz, C. Holland, and R.L. Jones. 2018. The Age-Friendly Community: A Test for Inclusivity. In *Age-Friendly Cities and Communities*, 251–272. Policy Press.

Rivera-Hernandez, M., A. Kumar, G. Epstein-Lubow, and K.S. Thomas. 2019. Disparities in Nursing Home Use and Quality Among African American, Hispanic, and White Medicare Residents with Alzheimer's Disease and Related Dementias. *Journal of Aging and Health* 31 (7): 1259–1277. https://doi.org/10.1177/0898264318767778.

Robert Wood Johnson Foundation. n.d. *Life Expectancy: Could Where You Live Influence How Long You Live?* RWJF. Retrieved March 21, 2023, from https://www.rwjf.org/en/insights/our-research/interactives/whereyouliveaffectshowlongyoulive.html

Sewell, A.A. 2016. Racism-Race Reification Process: A Mesolevel Political Economic Framework for Understanding Racial Health Disparities. *Sociology of Race and Ethnicity* 2 (4): 402–432.

Shippee, T.P., H. Davila, W. Ng, J.R. Bowblis, O. Akosionu, T. Skarphol, M.S. Thao, M. Woodhouse, and R.J. Thorpe. 2022. Evidence to Inform Policy and Practice: Mechanisms to Address Racial/Ethnic Disparities in Nursing Home Quality of Life. *Innovation in Aging* 6 (4): igac037. https://doi.org/10.1093/geroni/igac037.

Silva, A.D., T.E.D.C. Rosa, L.E. Batista, S. Kalckmann, M.C.P. Louvison, D.S.D.C. Teixeira, and M.L. Lebrão. 2019. Racial Inequities and Aging: Analysis of the 2010 Cohort of the Health, Welfare and Aging Study (SABE). *Revista Brasileira de Epidemiologia* 21 (Suppl 02): e180004. https://doi.org/10.1590/1980-549720180004.supl.2.

United Nations. 1982. *Report of the World Assembly on Ageing,* Vienna, 26 July–6 August. New York: United Nations.

———. 1999. *General Assembly President, Opening Assembly's Debate on Ageing, Says Theme of Year of Older Persons Founded on Inclusiveness.* UN Press. United Nations. Retrieved March 22, 2023, from https://press.un.org/en/1999/19991004.gasm106.doc.html

———. 2002. *Political Declaration and Madrid International Plan of Action on Ageing.* New York: United Nations. https://www.un.org/esa/socdev/documents/ageing/MIPAA/political-declaration-en.pdf

van Hoof, J., H.R. Marston, J.K. Kazak, and T. Buffel. 2021. Ten Questions Concerning Age-Friendly Cities and Communities and the Built Environment. *Building and Environment* 199: 107922.

Wallace, S. 2021. Health Inequities in Aging Adults from a Public Health Perspective. In *Oxford Research Encyclopedia of Global Public Health.*

WHO Commission on Social Determinants of Health, and World Health Organization 2008. *Closing the Gap in a Generation: Health Equity Through Action on the Social Determinants of Health – Final Report of the Commission on Social Determinants of Health.* World Health Organization.

Wilkinson, S., L. Lang, and S. Yarker. 2023. Dispersed Communities in Age-Friendly Work: An Intersectional Approach to Place-based Working. *Working with Older People* 27 (2): 110–119.

Willems, S.J., M.C. Castells, and A.P. Baptist. 2022. The Magnification of Health Disparities During the COVID-19 Pandemic. *The Journal of Allergy and Clinical Immunology: In Practice* 10 (4): 903–908.

Woolrych, R., J. Sixsmith, J. Duvvuru, A. Portella, M.L. Fang, D. Menezes, J. Henderson, J. Fisher, and R. Lawthom. 2022. Cross-National Perspectives on Aging and Place: Implications for Age-Friendly Cities and Communities. *The Gerontologist* 62 (1): 119–129.

World Health Organization. 2007. *Global Age-Friendly Cities: A Guide.* https://apps.who.int/iris/bitstream/handle/10665/43755/9789241547307_eng.pdf?sequence=1&isAll

———. n.d.. https://extranet.who.int/agefriendlyworld/age-friendly-cities-framework/

Chapter 3
Age-Friendly Neighborhoods

Andy Hong

Introduction

As the global population ages, there is an increasing need for age-friendly neighborhoods to support older adults to age in place. Aging in place refers to the ability of older adults to remain in their own homes and communities for as long as possible, with the necessary support and services to maintain their quality of life. In contrast, assisted living or nursing home facilities can be expensive and may not provide the same level of independence and autonomy as aging in place. While assisted living facilities can provide necessary care and support for older adults, they may not meet the needs and preferences of all older adults. A recent national survey reported that many older adults want to remain in their own homes and communities as long as they can (Robinson-Lane et al. 2022). Aging in place reduces the demand for institutionalized care, allowing people to maintain control over their environment and live more independently. Furthermore, doing so allows older people to maintain close ties with their families and communities.

Despite the growing demand for it, there are many challenges to aging in place. First, most homes are not designed with older adults in mind, lacking age-friendly features, such as single-story layouts, wider doorways, and accessible bathrooms (Forsyth et al. 2019). These age-friendly features are woven into the principles of universal design, which is aimed at creating environments, products, and services that cater to the diverse needs of individuals, regardless of age, fostering inclusivity and accessibility. Yet, the percentage of new housing units designed to universal design standards remains at 1 percent (Gentile 2017). In home care settings, many older adults may also face mobility challenges due to physical limitations or health

A. Hong (✉)
Healthy Aging and Resilient Places Lab, Department of City and Metropolitan Planning, College of Architecture + Planning, The University of Utah, Salt Lake City, UT, USA
e-mail: a.hong@utah.edu

V. Chang Greer, L. S. Edelman (eds.), *Age-Friendly Ecosystems*, SpringerBriefs in Public Health, https://doi.org/10.1007/978-3-031-68361-9_3

conditions, making it difficult to navigate their homes and communities. Inadequate transportation options can further limit mobility, making it challenging for older adults to access essential services and social activities. Furthermore, it can be expensive to retrofit homes with age-friendly features, which makes it challenging for low-income older adults to age in place.

The challenges of aging in place can be overcome by creating age-friendly neighborhoods. The concept of age-friendly neighborhood is rooted in the World Health Organization's Age-Friendly Cities and Communities initiative, which aims to create physical and social environments that support healthy aging and enable older adults to age in place (World Health Organization 2007). Age-friendly neighborhoods are characterized by a range of features, including accessible and affordable housing, safe and reliable transportation options, well-maintained outdoor spaces, opportunities for social engagement and inclusion, and access to high-quality healthcare services. These features are designed to promote physical and mental well-being, facilitate social connections, and provide older adults with the support they need to maintain independence and autonomy as they age.

In this context, this chapter provides an overview of the key challenges of aging in place and how age-friendly neighborhoods can help address these challenges by creating environments that support older adults' ability to age in place successfully. A case study is drawn to demonstrate how a metric-based tool, such as the Walk Audit Toolkit, can be utilized to address various challenges related to accessibility and equity in these neighborhoods. The case study also highlights local collaborations and partnerships that take co-creation approaches to community engagement and design, with a focus on age-friendly neighborhoods. Additionally, the chapter addresses the unique challenges faced by rural communities, with some suggestions on how transportation and digital technologies can be leveraged to improve livability in rural locations. The chapter concludes by demonstrating the importance of co-creation approaches to community engagement and design in promoting equity and improving livability in age-friendly neighborhoods, regardless of their location.

Challenges of Aging in Place

There are several challenges associated with aging in place. One major challenge is the lack of accessible housing that meets the needs of older adults who want to age in place. There are less than 5 percent of homes in the United States that are adequately equipped with basic accessibility features, such as no-step entry, single-floor living, wide doorways, and accessible electrical controls (Forsyth et al. 2019). Furthermore, even when these features are present, they may not be sufficient to meet the needs of individuals with disabilities or mobility impairments. Universal design, which involves designing buildings and spaces that are accessible to people of all ages and abilities, is essential for promoting accessibility and mobility for older adults. However, only 1 percent of new housing units are designed to meet universal design standards (Gentile 2017). The lack of accessible housing can have significant consequences for older adults. Without accessible features, older adults may be at risk of falls, which can result in serious injury and increased healthcare costs. In addition, the lack of accessibility can limit older adults' ability to perform daily activities, which could lead to social isolation and a lower quality of life.

Another major challenge of aging in place is housing affordability, particularly for those who are renters. According to a recent report, nearly one-third of households were "rent-burdened" in 2020, meaning they spent more than 30 percent of their income on housing costs (Joint Center for Housing Studies 2020). In addition, the report notes that the number of severely cost-burdened households, where housing costs exceed 50 percent of income, is about 14 percent (Joint Center for Housing Studies 2020). The high cost of housing is especially challenging for people who want to age in place. Many older people have fixed incomes that may not keep up with rising housing costs. In fact, more than half of all renters aged 65 and older are considered rent-burdened, which could result in limited resources to cover other essential expenses, such as health care and food (Pew Charitable Trusts 2018). Furthermore, older adults may incur additional costs as a result of home modifications or home care services to support their aging needs. These characteristics may make it more difficult for older adults to stay in their homes and communities, increasing the risk of social isolation and poor health. Lack of affordable and accessible housing options can also lead to an increase in sheltered homelessness among older adults. A report from the US Department of Housing and Urban Development (Henry et al. 2022) reported that sheltered homelessness among older adults increased by 10 percent from 2007 to 2017. This indicates a lack of affordable and accessible housing options for older adults, particularly those with low incomes.

When it comes to mobility, older adults face bigger challenges when they need to travel outside of their homes. In urban areas with high-quality public transit services, older adults tend to utilize public transit more often, especially when facing financial constraints or having physical limitations for driving. However, older adults in rural areas have limited mobility options and may need to rely on automobiles. While maintaining independent mobility through driving is important for older individuals, their safety is negatively impacted by physical frailty and cognitive impairment. These medical problems have varying effects on functional abilities needed for safe driving, such as risk perception and reaction time. As a result, promotion of old people's safe driving is vital, particularly given the high number of older adults who continue to drive with cognitive impairment. A recent study on older drivers in South Texas found that about 60 percent of older adults with mild cognitive impairment and 30 percent of older adults with dementia continue to drive (Malvitz et al. 2023). Older drivers sometimes fail to acknowledge or accept the decline in their driving abilities and their surrounding struggles with the conflict between maintaining their independence and mobility and the risk they bring to society and themselves.

Besides mobility, access to parks and healthy food options is also important for aging in place. However, disparities in access to these resources persist. Parks serving communities of color are often half the size of parks in predominantly white areas, limiting opportunities for physical activity and socialization (Trust for Public

Lands 2020). In addition, areas with limited access to affordable and healthy food options are significantly more abundant in minority neighborhoods (Bower et al. 2014). These disparities can negatively impact the health and well-being of older adults living in these communities.

Overall, the challenges of aging in place are significant and require comprehensive solutions that address affordability, mobility, accessibility, and access to resources such as housing, parks, and healthy food options. Age-friendly communities that prioritize the needs and preferences of older adults can play a crucial role in promoting successful aging in place.

Key Features of Age-Friendly Neighborhoods

Age-friendly neighborhoods are designed to provide physical, social, and emotional support to older adults, enabling them to age in place successfully. One of the most crucial aspects of age-friendly neighborhoods is housing, as a growing number of older adults want to stay in their homes as long as they can. Age-friendly neighborhoods can help make this possible by providing affordable, accessible, and adaptable housing options. Age-friendly neighborhoods should promote universal design principles that allow for the use and enjoyment of the built environment by people of all ages and abilities. This may include features such as step-free entrances, lever-style door handles, and non-slip flooring. Housing should also be affordable and accessible, with options for downsizing or shared living arrangements. Age-friendly neighborhoods can also provide resources to help older adults make modifications to their homes that will allow them to age in place safely and comfortably. Possible modifications may include adding features such as grab bars, wheelchair ramps, and wider doorways to accommodate mobility aids. In 2009, the Community Aging in Place—Advancing Better Living for Elders (CAPABLE) program began as a pilot study to leverage home modifications to increase older adults' daily function and independence. Since then, the CAPABLE program has been expanded, with more than 40 program sites across the country. A recent study has shown that the program offers significant benefits on a number of health-related outcomes, such as activities of daily living (ADL) limitations, fall efficacy, depression, and pain (Breysse et al. 2022).

Intergenerational living arrangements, where individuals of different ages cohabit, can be a means of addressing housing issues for both older adults and younger adults. Intergenerational living can provide older adults with companionship, assistance with daily duties, and support. It can provide affordable accommodation and a sense of community for young adults. There are a variety of intergenerational living arrangements, such as cohousing communities, shared living spaces, and family residences where older and younger adults reside together. These arrangements can be formal or informal and can be tailored to meet the specific needs of people involved. Intergenerational living arrangements can help break down age-related stereotypes and promote positive attitudes toward aging.

Intergenerational living can also facilitate mutual support between different age groups. For instance, younger individuals can provide older adults with practical assistance, such as assistance with transportation or domestic chores, whereas older adults can provide guidance and counsel based on their life experiences (Martinez et al. 2020). Moreover, intergenerational living can promote social interaction and combat social isolation. Sharing a living space with people of various ages can also provide opportunities for learning and personal development, as well as exposure to diverse perspectives and lifestyles.

Transportation is another critical aspect of age-friendly neighborhoods. Older adults who are no longer able to drive may face challenges accessing essential services and participating in community activities. Research has shown that driving cessation among older adults can have negative consequences on their quality of life, social connections, and overall health (Chihuri et al. 2016). Driving cessation can also lead to a decrease in social engagement and community participation, resulting in feelings of isolation and loneliness (Qin et al. 2020). To support older adults in their transition to later life, it is crucial to provide a range of transportation options that cater to their diverse needs. Such options can include accessible public transportation, community-based transportation services, and ride-hailing services that are affordable and easy to use. Providing such options can help older adults maintain their independence, social connections, and overall well-being. In addition to transportation options, age-friendly communities should also prioritize walkability, accessibility, and safety to promote physical activity and social engagement among older adults. These features can include well-maintained sidewalks, pedestrian crossings, benches, and public restrooms.

The outdoor environment is also an essential aspect of age-friendly neighborhoods. Accessible and well-maintained public spaces such as parks and green spaces can provide opportunities for outdoor activities such as gardening, walking, and other recreational activities. These activities have been shown to have physical and mental health benefits, including reducing the risk of chronic disease and improving mood (Coventry et al. 2021). In creating these spaces, public spaces should be designed with features that consider the physical and sensory abilities of older adults. For instance, providing seating, shade, and accessible restrooms can facilitate outdoor activities among older adults with mobility and balance issues. Proper lighting is also crucial to ensure visibility and reduce the risk of falls among older adults. In addition to promoting physical activity and social interaction, age-friendly neighborhoods can incorporate outdoor spaces that support the specific needs of older adults. For instance, community gardens and urban farms can provide opportunities for older adults to engage in meaningful activities, such as growing their food and engaging in intergenerational learning opportunities. Furthermore, outdoor spaces can be designed to support older adults' health needs, such as providing areas for relaxation and stress reduction, or outdoor fitness equipment tailored to older adults' needs.

Access to health care is an important factor in promoting healthy aging and supporting older adults to remain in their homes. With advancing age, individuals' healthcare needs become more complex and require more attention. Research shows that most older adults have one or more chronic diseases that require more frequent monitoring and treatment (Wolff et al. 2002). Therefore, age-friendly neighborhoods should prioritize the development of healthcare services and facilities that are accessible, affordable, and culturally appropriate for older adults. These services may include specialized clinics that cater to the specific healthcare needs of older adults, home healthcare services, and community health education programs.

In addition to ensuring access to health care, age-friendly neighborhoods should also support older adults to maintain their health and well-being. Physical activity is one of the most effective ways to promote health while preventing illness, disease, and frailty. However, over 80 percent of adults in the United States fail to meet the recommended guidelines (Elgaddal et al. 2022). Recent Centers for Disease Control and Prevention (CDC) data show that nearly 70 percent of adults over 75 report sitting for more than 8 h a day, and about 35 percent are entirely inactive (Elgaddal et al. 2022). This is concerning because sedentary lifestyles contribute to the early onset of illness. There is a dire need to stimulate regular physical activity at the population level. The built environment, particularly walkable neighborhoods, is one of the most powerful tools for promoting physical activity among older adults. Walkable neighborhoods are designed to make it easy and safe for residents to walk, bike, and use public transit. Typically, a mix of land uses, including shops, restaurants, and enterprises, are located within walking distance of one another. They also have sidewalks, crosswalks, and other amenities that make walking safer and more convenient. Research has shown that older adults who lived in walkable neighborhoods were more likely to be physically active than those who lived in car-dependent neighborhoods (Barnett et al. 2017). This is because walkable communities offer more opportunities for physical activity, such as walking to the store, the park, or the doctor. In addition, walkable neighborhoods can help reduce social isolation, which can be a significant problem among older adults.

Advancing Equity Through Community-Engaged Design

In creating age-friendly neighborhoods, it is important to incorporate principles of equity across all stages of development. One viable strategy for promoting equity is to actively engage the community in the planning and design phases (American Institute of Architects 2020). Community-engaged design brings together residents, local organizations, planners, and other stakeholders to collectively envision and cocreate age-friendly neighborhoods. This participatory approach allows for a deeper understanding of the specific challenges and aspirations of older adults within the community. By actively involving them in the decision-making process, their voices are heard, and their insights contribute to solutions that are both relevant and impactful. Through community-engaged design, older adults become not just beneficiaries but active contributors to the design of their living environment. They provide invaluable insights into the barriers they face, the amenities they require, and the social dynamics they seek. This inclusive process ensures that age-friendly solutions are tailored to the unique context and character of the neighborhood.

Moreover, community engagement serves as a catalyst for social cohesion and strengthens intergenerational bonds. It creates opportunities for different age groups to interact, share experiences, and learn from one another. In this way, age-friendly neighborhoods become spaces where the collective wisdom of older adults is integrated with the innovative perspectives of younger generations, enriching the overall fabric of the community. Engaging the community in the design process not only enhances the physical aspects of walkability but also cultivates a sense of ownership and pride among residents. This sense of ownership translates to a commitment to maintaining and nurturing the age-friendly features of the neighborhood, ensuring their sustainability over time. The case study shown in Box 3.1 is a powerful illustration of how individuals with a strong commitment may collaborate, transcend divergences, and strive toward a collective objective of fostering inclusive and dynamic neighborhoods that cater to people of all ages.

In essence, community-engaged design amplifies the principles of equity, inclusivity, and social connection in the creation of age-friendly, walkable neighborhoods. It elevates the voices of older adults, recognizes their expertise, and transforms them into cocreators of vibrant, accessible, and thriving communities that benefit everyone.

Box 3.1: Case Study: Bridging Communities Through the State Walking College Program

The Walking College, launched by America Walks in 2015, aimed to empower local advocates in creating livable, walkable communities across the United States (America Walks 2023). Over the course of 8 years, the program facilitated skills training for 180 Walking College Fellows, fostering a network of peer experts and the implementation of localized Walking Action Plans. This case study focuses on the State Walking College program's impact on two neighboring communities, Marin City and Sausalito, in California. Marin City and Sausalito, separated by US Highway 101, historically faced disparities driven by racial injustice. While Marin City's population is predominantly Black and Hispanic with a median age of 40, Sausalito is about 90 percent white, older (55 years), and wealthier.

The State Walking College provided an opportunity to address these disparities and bring these communities together. Juanita Edwards, Sybil Boutilier, and Vicki Nichols, representing Marin City and Sausalito, engaged in community healing efforts prior to their involvement in the State Walking College. Recognizing the potential for inclusivity, Sybil formed a team with Vicki and Juanita to participate in the program. Their joint vision aimed to create safer and more inviting walking and biking spaces across both communities by developing the Walking Action Plan focused on inter-community and intergenerational activities. Partnering with the merged Sausalito/Marin City School District and the County's Safe Routes to School program, they aimed to establish Walking School Buses, Social Walking Groups, and a

Box 3.1 (continued)
"Safe Walking and Biking" Education Program. They also advocated for street and sidewalk improvements, utilizing the Walk Audit Tool Kit by the American Association of Retired Persons (AARP).

Since completing the State Walking College program, the Sausalito/Marin City team has achieved several milestones. Some of the tangible results include (1) launching a Bike Safety Program in collaboration with Marin County; (2) promoting pedestrian and bicycle safety messaging through community events and social media; (3) engaging advisory roles with the Marin County Transit Authority; (4) advocating for the renewal of a sales tax measure supporting trail improvements; and (5) contributing to the installation of a mural connecting the two communities. The success of the Sausalito/Marin City team can be attributed to community engagement, active listening, and empathy. Vicki emphasized the importance of not imposing solutions but rather collaborating with partners and communities to achieve meaningful change.

Overall, the State Walking College program facilitated by America Walks and AARP Livable Communities has proven its potential to bridge communities, address historical disparities, and create tangible improvements in walkability. The collaboration between Juanita, Sybil, and Vicki serves as a compelling example of how dedicated individuals can come together, overcome differences, and work toward a shared vision of inclusiveness and vibrant, age-friendly neighborhoods.

Age-Friendly Neighborhoods in Rural Communities

Older adults in rural communities face a unique set of challenges, including limited access to services, resources, and social activities. These challenges can have a significant impact on the health and well-being of older adults, and they can make it difficult for them to age in place. One of the most significant challenges faced by older adults in rural areas is the limited access to healthcare facilities and specialized medical services. Rural communities tend to have a scarcity of healthcare professionals, medical facilities, and transportation options. This lack of healthcare access can lead to delayed or inadequate medical attention, making it difficult for older adults to manage chronic health conditions effectively. Isolation is another major challenge for older adults in rural communities. Rural communities are often more sparsely populated than urban areas, which means that there are fewer opportunities for older adults to connect with friends, family, and community members. Rural communities often have fewer social services and transportation options, which can make it difficult for older adults to get out and about and meet new people. The lack of adequate transportation options for older adults further increases isolation in rural communities. Unlike urban areas with abundant public transportation options, rural areas often face significant challenges in providing adequate transportation services to meet the needs of older residents. Therefore, most older adults in rural areas rely on their private automobiles to get to places. This leaves them with few transportation options when they get older and need to stop driving due to health concerns.

One important way to make rural areas more age-friendly is to improve transportation options. This includes providing on-demand transportation services, such as Via and autonomous shuttles. On-demand transportation services are similar to Uber or Lyft, but they use vehicles that are ADA compliant. Autonomous shuttles are driverless vehicles that are being piloted in several cities across the United States (Haque and Brakewood 2020). In addition to improving transportation options, digital technologies can be used to provide older adults with access to healthcare services, educational opportunities, and social activities. They can also be used to connect older adults with their families and friends who live in other parts of the country or the world. For example, telemedicine can be a valuable tool for older adults in rural areas. These areas often have limited access to healthcare providers, and telemedicine can help to bridge the gap. Telemedicine can also help to reduce the cost of health care for older adults, as they may not have to travel long distances to see a doctor. Telemedicine can also help improve the quality of care as it offers greater access to specialists and makes it easier for rural patients to see their doctors for routine visits. Together with improvement in transportation, digital technologies have the potential to make a significant impact on the lives of older adults and create more age-friendly environments in rural communities.

Conclusion

The desire among older adults to age in place is strong; however, this aspiration is often hindered by a number of challenges associated with lack of age-friendly infrastructure at the neighborhood scale. The prevalent lack of age-friendly features in many homes, compounded by mobility obstacles and inadequate transportation choices, underscores the pressing need for transformative change in urban and rural communities. In response to these challenges, the concept of age-friendly neighborhoods emerges as a viable solution. These neighborhoods are designed to promote physical, social, and emotional support, offering older adults the opportunity to age well while remaining in familiar surroundings. Central to the success of age-friendly neighborhoods are housing, transportation, and outdoor environments, which collectively create an ecosystem that nurtures and sustains independent living.

One key aspect of age-friendly neighborhoods is the principle of walkability. Illustrated by the collaborative efforts between America Walks and AARP, the potential of walkable communities extends far beyond meeting the needs of older adults. The concept serves as a blueprint for designing neighborhoods that prioritize the well-being and connectivity of all residents. By integrating universal design principles into the fabric of walkability, neighborhoods can further embrace diversity, ensuring accessibility for individuals of all ages and abilities.

In rural communities, the challenges faced by older adults take on a unique dimension, one that requires tailored solutions to ensure their ability to age in place with dignity and vitality. The transformative power of age-friendly neighborhoods holds significant promise for rural areas as well, with improved transportation options emerging as a pivotal strategy. Initiatives like on-demand transportation services and autonomous shuttles can bridge the geographic gaps that often isolate older adults in rural settings.

In conclusion, creating age-friendly neighborhoods is a community-wide effort that benefits everyone. By prioritizing inclusive housing, accessible transportation, welcoming outdoor spaces, and thoughtful urban design, we can build vibrant communities where older adults thrive and all residents enjoy a higher quality of life. This approach not only fosters a strong sense of belonging but also demonstrates the importance of equiatable and inclusive planning and design. Age-friendly neighborhoods offers as a powerful place-based strategy that enables everyone to feel valued and live fulfilling lives.

References

America Walks. 2023. *Stories from the State Walking College: An Idea Book for Taking Action to Create More Walkable Communities*. America Walks. https://aw2021.wpenginepowered.com/wp-content/uploads/2023/01/Final-Report-Stories-from-the-Walking-College.pdf

American Institute of Architects. 2020. *Engaging Community*. Guides for Equitable Practice. https://www.aia.org/pages/6253015-engaging-community

Barnett, D.W., A. Barnett, A. Nathan, J. Van Cauwenberg, and E. Cerin. 2017. Built Environmental Correlates of Older Adults' Total Physical Activity and Walking: A Systematic Review and Meta-Analysis. *International Journal of Behavioral Nutrition and Physical Activity* 14 (1): 1–24. https://doi.org/10.1186/s12966-017-0558-z.

Bower, K.M., R.J. Thorpe Jr., C. Rohde, and D.J. Gaskin. 2014. The Intersection of Neighborhood Racial Segregation, Poverty, and Urbanicity and Its Impact on Food Store Availability in the United States. *Preventive Medicine* 58: 33–39. https://doi.org/10.1016/j.ypmed.2013.10.010.

Breysse, J., S. Dixon, J. Wilson, and S. Szanton. 2022. Aging Gracefully in Place: An Evaluation of the Capability of the CAPABLE© Approach. *Journal of Applied Gerontology* 41 (3): 718–728. https://doi.org/10.1177/07334648211042606.

Chihuri, S., T.J. Mielenz, C.J. DiMaggio, M.E. Betz, C. DiGuiseppi, V.C. Jones, and G. Li. 2016. Driving Cessation and Health Outcomes in Older Adults. *Journal of the American Geriatrics Society* 64 (2): 332–341. https://doi.org/10.1111/jgs.13931.

Coventry, P.A., J.E. Brown, J. Pervin, S. Brabyn, R. Pateman, J. Breedvelt, S. Gilbody, R. Stancliffe, R. McEachan, and P.L. White. 2021. Nature-based Outdoor Activities for Mental and Physical Health: Systematic Review and Meta-Analysis. *SSM: Population Health* 16: 100934. https://doi.org/10.1016/j.ssmph.2021.100934.

Elgaddal, N., E.A. Kramarow, and C. Reuben. 2022. Physical Activity Among Adults Aged 18 and Over: United States, 2020. *NCHS Data Brief* no. 443. Hyattsville, MD: National Center for Health Statistics. https://doi.org/10.15620/cdc:120213.

Forsyth, A., J. Molinsky, and H.Y. Kan. 2019. Improving Housing and Neighborhoods for the Vulnerable: Older People, Small Households, Urban Design, and Planning. *Urban Design International* 24: 171–186. https://doi.org/10.1057/s41289-019-00081-x.

Gentile, A. 2017. Will Your Home Be Ready for Aging in Place? *Forbes*. Retrieved May 17, 2023. https://www.forbes.com/sites/nextavenue/2017/05/03/will-your-home-be-ready-for-aging-in-place

Haque, A.M., and C. Brakewood. 2020. A Synthesis and Comparison of American Automated Shuttle Pilot Projects. *Case Studies on Transport Policy* 8 (3): 928–937.

Henry, M., T. de Sousa, T. Baker, J. Cusick, R. Hull, and J. Marson. 2022. The 2019–2020 Annual Homeless Assessment Report (AHAR) to Congress. US Department of Housing and Urban Development. https://www.huduser.gov/portal/datasets/ahar/2020-ahar-part-2-pit-estimates-of-homelessness-in-the-us.html

Joint Center for Housing Studies. 2020. *The State of the Nation's Housing*. Harvard University. https://www.jchs.harvard.edu/state-nations-housing-2020

Malvitz, M., D.B. Zahuranec, W. Chang, S.G. Heeringa, E.M. Briceño, R. Mehdipanah, X.F. Gonzales, D.A. Levine, K.M. Langa, N. Garcia, and L.B. Morgenstern. 2023. Driving Predictors in a Cohort of Cognitively Impaired Mexican American and Non-Hispanic White Individuals. *Journal of the American Geriatrics Society* 71: 3520. https://doi.org/10.1111/jgs.18493.

Martinez, L., R.M. Mirza, A. Austen, J. Hsieh, C.A. Klinger, M. Kuah, A. Liu, L. McDonald, R. Mohsin, C. Pang, J. Rajewski, T. Salomons, and I. Sheikh. 2020. More Than Just a Room: A Scoping Review of the Impact of Homesharing for Older Adults. *Innovation in Aging* 4 (2): igaa011. https://doi.org/10.1093/geroni/igaa011.

Pew Charitable Trusts. 2018. *American Families Face a Growing Rent Burden*. https://www.pewtrusts.org/-/media/assets/2018/04/rent-burden_report_v2.pdf

Qin, W., X. Xiang, and H. Taylor. 2020. Driving Cessation and Social Isolation in Older Adults. *Journal of Aging and Health* 32 (9): 962–971. https://doi.org/10.1177/0898264319870400.

Robinson-Lane, S. D., M. Singer, E. Kirch, E. Solway, J. Smith, J. Kullgren, and P. Malani. 2022. *Older Adults' Preparedness to Age in Place*. University of Michigan National Poll on Healthy Aging. Retrieved May 23, 2023. https://doi.org/10.7302/4278.

Trust for Public Lands. 2020. *The Heat Is On: A Trust for Public Land Special Report*. https://www.tpl.org/wp-content/uploads/2022/09/The-Heat-is-on_A-Trust-for-Public-Land_special-report.pdf

Wolff, J.L., B. Starfield, and G. Anderson. 2002. Prevalence, Expenditures, and Complications of Multiple Chronic Conditions in the Elderly. *Archives of Internal Medicine* 162 (20): 2269–2276. https://doi.org/10.1001/archinte.162.20.2269.

World Health Organization. 2007. *Global Age-Friendly Cities: A Guide*. World Health Organization: Geneva, Switzerland. https://apps.who.int/iris/handle/10665/43755

Chapter 4
Age-Friendly Campuses

Joann M. Montepare, Kimberly S. Farah, Lauren Marshall Bowen, Nina M. Silverstein, and Susan K. Whitbourne

The Need for Age-Friendly Campuses

Shifting age demographics are a defining issue of our time. Across the United States, communities are witnessing historic age shifts with the number of adults aged 65+ increasing annually as more individuals experience extended longevity. By 2030, the United States' older population will double in size, and one in five Americans

J. M. Montepare (✉)
Rosemary B. Fuss Center for Research on Aging and Intergenerational Studies, Lasell University, Newton, MA, USA
e-mail: jmontepare@lasell.edu

K. S. Farah
School of Health Sciences, Lasell University, Newton, MA, USA
e-mail: kfarah@lasell.edu

L. M. Bowen
Department of English, College of Liberal Arts, Gerontology Department and Institute, Manning College of Nursing and Health Sciences, University of Massachusetts Boston, Boston, MA, USA
e-mail: lauren.bowen@umb.edu

N. M. Silverstein
Gerontology Department and Institute, Manning College of Nursing and Health Sciences, University of Massachusetts Boston, Boston, MA, USA
e-mail: nina.silverstein@umb.edu

S. K. Whitbourne
Gerontology Department and Institute, Manning College of Nursing and Health Sciences, University of Massachusetts Boston, Boston, MA, USA

Department of Psychological and Brain Sciences; Gerontology Department and Institute, Manning College of Nursing and Health Sciences, University of Massachusetts Amherst, Boston, Boston, MA, USA
e-mail: susan.whitbourne@umb.edu

V. Chang Greer, L. S. Edelman (eds.), *Age-Friendly Ecosystems*, SpringerBriefs in Public Health, https://doi.org/10.1007/978-3-031-68361-9_4

will be over the age of 65, making our social structure more diverse than ever before (U.S. Census Bureau 2020).

Recognizing this demographic transformation, educators in the aging field have long called for institutions of higher education to prepare for the implications of increases in the older adult population (McGuire et al. 2005; Morrow-Howell et al. 2020; Sanchez and Kaplan 2014). The aging population is generating a rapidly growing longevity economy that will require a trained workforce to provide support services for the health and well-being of individuals as they age. Broader industry sectors that provide goods and experiences for an older consumer market in technology, travel, entertainment, home design, fashion, and more will also see growth (Coughlin 2017; Gerontological Society of America 2018). Thus, aging populations are creating career opportunities for students in higher education across diverse educational majors (Grawe 2018; Whitbourne and Montepare 2017).

Despite these developments, students are seldom taught about aging and rarely interact with older individuals in educational exchange. Thus, most will graduate with a negligible awareness of aging issues and the benefits of intergenerational connections. In turn, they will enter their personal and professional worlds lacking aging literacy and aging readiness (McGuire et al. 2005; Whitbourne and Montepare 2017). Moreover, the number of high-school graduates is declining and the population of young adults pursuing post-secondary education is shrinking, resulting in a demographic enrollment cliff with significant consequences for higher education (Grawe 2018). As a result, institutions will need to respond to the changing profile of students in higher education and reconsider distinctions between traditional (under 25 years) versus nontraditional students (over 25 years) (Sánchez and Kaplan 2014).

In contrast to a declining student population, a growing number of older adults are looking to higher education for educational opportunities to meet their professional needs as they experience longer work lives, move through multiple career paths, delay retirement, and continue to work for income and job advancement (Montepare 2019; Van Horn et al. 2015). Similarly, many adults plan to pursue some form of learning for personal development as they age (DiSilvestro 2013; Larkin et al. 2007). Over a decade ago, the American Council on Education (ACE) anticipated that many older adults would stay engaged in learning, work, or community service as they age (Larkin et al. 2007). Confirming this prediction, a later national survey by the Pew Research Center (2016) found that over 73 percent of older adults queried consider themselves to be "lifelong learners" and 74 percent were "personal learners" who engage in at least one formal activity annually to advance their knowledge (e.g., taking courses or attending events tied to learning).

The American Council on Education (Larkin et al. 2007) has questioned how institutions will adapt their programs, policies, and practices to meet the needs precipitated by emerging age-diverse, older populations. The Age-Friendly University (AFU) initiative provides one answer. The AFU initiative, launched in 2015, reflects the work of an international, interdisciplinary team of educators convened at Dublin City University, in collaboration with Arizona State University and the University of Strathclyde, to identify the specific ways campuses can respond to an aging population (O'Kelly 2015). The team articulated ten principles describing age-friendly educational practices (see Box 4.1) reflecting six pillars of institutional activity: teaching and learning, research and innovation, lifelong learning, intergenerational learning, encore careers and enterprise, and civic engagement.

The AFU principles advocate that older adults be enabled to participate in educational, career, cultural, and wellness activities on campuses, and that campuses extend aging education to younger students and abate age segregation by bringing younger and older learners together in educational exchange. In addition, age-friendly campuses support aging research informed by older adults' diverse needs and look to develop partnerships beyond their campuses with the local aging community (Montepare 2019).

The AFU network has grown from a few institutions to an international network of over 100 campuses in Europe, North America, South America, and Asia. Momentum to build the network continues, with the endorsement of professional

Box 4.1: Ten Principles for an Age-Friendly University (AFU)

1. To encourage the participation of older adults in all the *core activities* of the university, including educational and research programs.
2. To promote personal and career development in the second half of life and to support those who wish to pursue *second careers*.
3. To recognize the *range of educational needs* of older adults (from those who were early school-leavers through to those who wish to pursue Master's or PhD qualifications).
4. To promote *intergenerational learning* to facilitate the reciprocal sharing of expertise between learners of all ages.
5. To widen access to *online educational opportunities* for older adults to ensure a diversity of routes to participation.
6. To ensure that the university's *research agenda* is informed by the needs of an aging society and to promote public discourse on how higher education can better respond to the varied interests and needs of older adults.
7. To increase the understanding of students of the *longevity dividend* and the increasing complexity and richness that aging brings to our society.
8. To enhance access for older adults to the university's range of *health and wellness* programs and its *arts* and *cultural activities*.
9. To engage actively with the university's own *retired community*.
10. To ensure regular *dialogue* with organizations representing the interests of the aging population.

Source: Reprinted with permission from Age-Friendly University Global Network (n.d.). https://www.afugn.org/principles

organizations such as the Gerontological Society of America (GSA) and its Academy for Gerontology in Higher Education (AGHE). Moreover, the AFU initiative joins other leading-edge initiatives that share the common goal of moving toward a global age-friendly ecosystem, including age-friendly communities, age-friendly health systems, and age-friendly employers, all of which offer collaborative opportunities for age-friendly campuses, which we describe below (Fulmer et al. 2020).

In addition to being a learning environment central to the educational needs of an age-diverse population, higher education is also a natural work environment where faculty and staff are "aging in place in the workplace" (Silverstein et al. 2021). Currently, the median age of all employees in higher education is older than the overall median US workforce. Moreover, US higher education already has more older employees than the projected 25 percent labor force share forecasted for 2024 (Pritchard et al. 2019). These statistics further signal the need for institutions to examine how they can support employees as they move through their work lives in academia and the many aging-related experiences they will encounter along the way.

As aging-supportive learning and work environments, age-friendly campuses also reflect beneficial pathways for aging. Considerable empirical studies have shown the positive benefits of cognitive engagement. For instance, a review of the adult development and aging literature conducted by Hertzog et al. (2008) supported the hypothesis that an active lifestyle and cognitive engagement promote healthy aging. In their review of the relationship between education and well-being, Lövdén et al. (2020) further showed that the number of years of education one completed is positively correlated with one's cognitive function throughout adulthood and predicts a lower dementia risk later in life. Thus, engaging in lifelong learning that age-friendly campuses can provide is critical to the health and well-being of individuals as they age. Indeed, adults surveyed by the Pew Research Center who engaged in learning activities reported psychological and social rewards (Park et al. 2014). Specifically, participating made them feel more capable and well-rounded, and the learning experience presented new perspectives, forged new friendships, and made local community connections. Experimental research has supported self-reported positive outcomes. Using a modified random-control design, Lenehan et al. (2016) found that older adults who took college courses showed a significant increase in their cognitive capacity (an identified dementia predictor) in comparison to a control group of peers who did not take courses. Although no research to date has examined the benefits of working in an age-friendly campus environment, research looking at the benefits of age-friendly workplaces can easily be applied to campus settings (Eppler-Hattab et al. 2020).

The Need for Empirical Tools and Approaches

Age-friendly campuses can advance educational practices in a variety of ways that align with AFU principles and make for more supportive work environments through other practices. However, doing so challenges institutions to assess existing programs, assess perceptions of campus members, and develop plans to address gaps and opportunities (Clark and Leedahl 2019; Simon et al. 2020). Some researchers have begun to examine age-friendly campus efforts using surveys of leaders at AFU campuses or interviews of stakeholders in select campus divisions (Lim et al. 2022; Simon et al. 2020). Others have used photovoice strategies that use photographs taken by selected participants and their evaluations of the images to evaluate physical supports and barriers (Chesser et al. 2020) and focus groups to assess the needs of older students with respect to specific functions, such as admissions and career services (Morrow-Howell et al. 2022. Although informative, more comprehensive approaches are needed to evaluate campus-wide practices that impact not only students but also faculty and staff. Additionally, measures are needed that consider the perceptions of these practices by campus community members.

Using a systems-level, campus-wide lens, the Age-Friendly Inventory and Campus Climate Survey (ICCS) was recently developed by Silverstein et al. (2021), which campuses can use to evaluate both the nature of age-friendly practices and the perceptions of these practices by students, faculty, and staff. The design of the ICCS is based on the concept of person-environment fit within the context of a social-ecological model articulated by Moos and Moos (1983). According to this model, the quality of an individual's adaptation and advantage in an environment will depend on the match between the actual and the ideal or expected components of the environment. As such, the ICCS assesses the "objective" features of a campus environment reflected in existing age-friendly practices with an inventory of 93 possible practices across seven core institutional functions (see Table 4.1: Age-friendly inventory): community outreach and engagement, personnel, physical environment, research, services, student affairs, and teaching and learning.

Table 4.1 Age-friendly inventory

Function	Practices
Community outreach and engagement	Intergenerational opportunities; services, events, and other discounts for retirees/older adults in the community; retired faculty/staff associations
Personnel	Mentoring and professional development; preretirement planning; events to recognize longstanding employees
Physical environment	Visible signage, minimized walking distances, accessible bathrooms, hallways well-lit and free of obstacles, handicapped parking, and maps and communication systems for navigation
Research	Support for aging-related research; opportunities for collaboration and funding, dissemination of findings
Services	Caregiving support and services; other services for older students and employees including health care, fitness and wellness, and technology support
Student affairs	Services for older students including career services, recruiting, admissions, orientations, and opportunities to join campus organizations
Teaching and learning	Student academic support services; courses with aging content; availability of support and funding for new aging-focused courses; lifelong learning opportunities

Source: Silverstein et al. (2021)

The “subjective” features of the environment, or how individuals view and experience these practices, are assessed with a Campus Climate Survey. A computed “match” score component reflects the extent to which practices align with perceptions and evaluates if there was a particular practice in place, were campus members aware of it, and did they value such practices.

In a study using the ICCS across a sample of 20 diverse AFU institutions in the United States, demographic data revealed that contrary to the common conception of higher education as being an age-segregated environment, campuses are indeed age-diverse communities (Montepare 2021). More specifically, across institutions, 19 percent of campus members were under the age of 24 years, 30 percent were 25–44 years, 18 percent were 45–54 years, 21 percent were 55–64 years, and 13 percent were 65 years and older. Considerable variation was also seen across campus functions in the extent to which age-friendly practices were in place. The highest overall ICCS score obtained for a campus was the existence of 77 out of 93 age-friendly practices, but the mean scores across all campuses were only about 65 percent. The campus function that received the highest scores fell into the category of those concerning the physical environment, likely reflecting external accountability such as the required Americans with Disability Act mandates. In contrast, overall scores for campus functions in teaching and learning, research, and community outreach and engagement were much lower, with scores for services and resources, personnel, and student affairs being somewhat higher. Thus, gaps are especially evident (even on AFU campuses) with respect to aging education, aging research, and community connections, as well as with academic and career support for older learners, faculty, and staff. Research is now needed to understand the nature of best practices in these areas and how campuses can design and implement practical, feasible, and impactful strategies to expand their age-friendly efforts.

More revealing, extremely low ICCS match scores showed that even for campuses reporting a relatively high number of age-friendly practices being in place, the constituents who study and work on the campuses and would benefit from them were generally unaware that the practices existed. Finally, overall perceptions of the age-friendliness of a campus were predicted by the match between practices and perceptions of those campuses. Individuals who were aware of various age-friendly campus practices perceived their campus to be more age-friendly. The latter findings suggest more broadly that age inclusivity means moving beyond the mere presence of age-friendly practices and includes how these practices are valued, recognized, and integrated into the campus mission, infrastructure, and curriculum.

In addition to providing a deeper understanding of the nature of age inclusivity in higher education, findings from ICCS research suggest several actions institutions should consider beyond the implementation of AFU principles and related practices. One is that any age-friendly campus initiative should build in opportunities to make campus members aware of the reasons why being more age inclusive is important, along with opportunities to raise awareness about the nature of ongoing and planned age-friendly programs and policies. Mounting more age-friendly practices also will require professional development opportunities and incentives geared toward engaging faculty and campus leaders around age-inclusive best practices in teaching, research, and community engagement. Institutions also need to consider ways to make aging education more accessible in the curriculum and to integrate age inclusivity in broader diversity, equity, and inclusion efforts. Additionally, the view of higher education as being an age-segregated environment needs to be revised to recognize age-diverse faculty and staff members who would benefit from more age-friendly organizational workplace practices.

Future empirical studies will be needed to extend existing research. In particular, research is needed to examine in more detail not only strategies for long-term engagement but also structural barriers that constrain some older individuals from pursuing educational opportunities on age-friendly campuses (Richards 2020). For example, campuses may offer coursework in topics of interest to older individuals but fail to consider issues related to accessibility, such as remote technology and transportation, that may make it challenging for some to participate in these programs. Such problems are particularly acute for individuals who have limited access to technology or have health restrictions that prohibit them from engaging virtually or in person with campus offerings. Moreover, these barriers may create further disparities for particular populations of older adults. Hansen et al. (2019) found in their study of lifelong learning programs that the representation of older learners from racial and ethnic minority groups was limited in comparison to other groups participating in higher education programs. Furthermore, there is an underrepresentation of individuals who have not attained bachelor's level degrees, as well as individuals for whom time and cost are concerns. Thus, research is needed to understand the structural barriers to access as well as the personal factors that contribute to the low engagement of some older individuals.

The Need to Build Age-Friendly Ecosystem Connections

Fulmer et al. (2020) describe how the age-friendly construct has expanded to include campuses, cities, states, countries, businesses, healthcare systems, and public health systems following the introduction of the Global Network for Age-Friendly Cities and Communities (AFCC) initiative by the World Health Organization (WHO) in 2002. They also point out that beyond merely constructing independent age-friendly environments, there is a fundamental need to build connections across them to inform the respective efforts. Of equal importance, the sustainability of age-friendly initiatives will be enhanced by "spillover" effects, in which behavioral or policy efforts in one environment spur action and change in another environment (Coyle et al. 2022).

Examples of such synergy can be seen in collaborations between AFUs and AFCCs in which institutions have provided expertise and support to facilitate the development of community action plans (Luz and Baldwin 2019). Faculty and students from Portland State University helped to develop procedures to assess the meaning of age-friendliness and age-friendly community needs that informed strategic planning and policy decisions with project leaders and community members in the city of Portland (Neal et al. 2014). Similarly, the University of Massachusetts Boston provided vital support to diverse age-friendly communities in the greater Boston area not only by designing and implementing community-wide evaluation strategies but also by generating demographic and health profiles (Healthy Aging Data Reports) that provide accurate, unbiased local community and statewide information about aging data (Dugan et al. 2022). Such collaborative town-gown partnerships are especially impactful when community efforts are challenged by limited resources and the need for experts in aging to inform the evaluation, design, and implementation of age-friendly efforts (Filinson and Raimondo 2019).

AFU programs tailored to specific community partnerships also demonstrate how age-friendly campuses can contribute to the ability of AFCCs to provide support and resources within the eight WHO domains of livability (Outdoor Spaces and Buildings, Transportation, Housing, Social Participation, Respect and Social Inclusion, Work and Civic Engagement, Communication and Information, Community and Health Services). For example, the AgeAlive program at Michigan State University maintains a database of aging-related research, courses, outreach programs, and service organizations on campus and in the surrounding communities (Luz and Baldwin 2019). The MedEx Wellness program hosted at Dublin City University offers a community-based chronic disease exercise rehabilitation program to support physical, clinical, and psychological health (Kehoe et al. 2020). The University of Rhode Island developed an intergenerational service-learning reverse mentoring program in which students helped older community members learn about technology—enhancing both social participation and skill building (Leedahl et al. 2018). Along similar lines, the University of Akron mounted a collaborative research effort between researchers on aging and a government-sponsored program to provide learning opportunities for older adults and engagement for individuals with developmental disabilities (Stanley et al. 2019). Central Connecticut State University's Scholars for Life! provided engagement opportunities for older community members through a faculty guest lecture series (June and Andreoletti 2023). During the COVID-19 pandemic, participation swelled via a virtual delivery option, showing how AFUs can serve important roles in navigating needs brought about by crises in communities.

It is also of interest to consider how collaborations with local communities can help to inform age-friendly campus efforts. For example, AFU institutions have gathered input from local community members to understand barriers and supports to their campus age-friendliness and to guide strategic planning around age-friendly initiatives (Cannon et al. 2021; Chesser et al. 2020). Colorado University Anschutz Medical Campus has developed an innovative program in which Older Adult Research Specialists (OARS) from the local community join campus research teams to serve as local experts for education, recruitment, and retainment of older adults in research and clinical trials (Meyer 2022).

Another pioneering program that complements the AFU initiative is the Age-Friendly Health System (AFHS) program developed by the John A. Hartford Foundation, the Institute for Healthcare Improvement, the American Hospital Association, and the Catholic Health Association of the United States (Fulmer et al.

2020; De Biasi et al. 2020). The AFHS model uses four evidence-based elements, collectively referred to as the 4Ms (What Matters, Medication, Mentation, Mobility) to guide the delivery of healthcare to older adults. Dialogue and collaborations between AFUs and AFHSs would help to support each initiative's endeavors as well as strengthen and amplify new and ongoing activities. For example, faculty and graduate students on the AFU University of Maryland campus volunteered to teach and mentor hospital staff on 4 M projects: (1) Get to Know Me Boards filled by staff caring for hospitalized older adults (Matters); (2) Medical Intensive Care Unit discharge opioid medication deprescribing (Medication); and (3) UMove Mobility (Schumacher et al. 2022).

AFU-AFHS partnerships are poised to inspire new research initiatives and clinical programs, encourage the participation of older adults in the development and evaluation of these efforts, and promote public discourse on how higher education and medical systems can better respond to the diverse needs of older adults. Systemic disparities could also be addressed. For example, minoritized older adults often do not trust that physicians will fully explain research programs and are therefore reluctant to participate in them (Corbie-Smith et al. 2002). Experts on aging at AFUs could help to remedy this mistrust by playing a leadership role in educating physicians about effective communication strategies. They could also steer discussions with older adults about how historical harms and discriminatory actions of current health systems can be improved through their research participation. A community participatory approach facilitated by experts on AFU campuses could be used to develop action plans during community crises such as the COVID-19 pandemic, illuminate best practices, and ensure that older adults have a voice in developing ethical and effective health practices (Montepare and Brown 2022).

AFUs could also join forces with businesses that are members of the Age-Friendly Employer (AFE) initiative (https://institute.agefriendly.org), which certifies employers as "age-friendly" in recognition of their commitment to valuing employees based not on their age, but on their proficiencies, qualifications, and contributions. To qualify as an AFE, current policies, practices, and programs should be aligned with providing older employees aged 50 and above with meaningful employment, developmental opportunities, competitive pay, and benefits. To this end, AFUs could offer age-friendly employers educational opportunities for their older employees, as well as pipelines for younger employees who appreciate age diversity and understand the value of older adults' knowledge, maturity, reliability, and productivity in the workplace.

Many AFEs represent aging-related organizations that are facing a high demand for practitioners with expertise in aging (Moye et al. 2019). AFU-AFE partnerships could respond in several ways. For example, AFUs could mount more age-friendly health professions and related education programs, along with career support incentives, at the undergraduate, graduate, and postgraduate levels that would address demand by building stronger educational pipelines (Gugliucci and O'Neil 2019). An important component of mounting pathways for careers in the aging field is providing students and emerging professionals with opportunities for aging-based internships, practicums, or field placements alongside opportunities for employment (Karasik et al. 2022). AFEs in the aging sector could help to create these opportunities in collaboration with AFUs.

It is clear that age-friendly campuses have a great deal to offer in their own right as well as in connection with other age-friendly initiatives. However, it is important to consider ways in which AFU efforts and related campus initiatives will need to be improved and expanded. For example, the AFU framework could expand its principles beyond older learners to older faculty and staff who constitute core campus constituents. Deeper attention will need to be given to recognizing intersectionality and integrating age-inclusivity efforts with other diversity, inclusion, and equity efforts that are in motion on many campuses, which can be a challenging undertaking for a variety of reasons. Relatedly, age-friendly campus efforts will need to ensure they are inclusive across socioeconomic, racial, ethnic, and other social identity lines, lest disparities in educational access be inadvertently intensified. Moving forward, the broader AFU initiative also will need to navigate campuses that range in size, focus, location, and culture, along with addressing issues of organizational structure and information flow.

The Need to Dismantle Ageism

Proponents of the age-friendly ecosystem note its pivotal role in addressing the broader social issue of ageism (Fulmer et al. 2020). The case for more age-friendly campuses can also be made from the perspective of dismantling persistent ageism and its repercussions. Ageist beliefs permeate society with age stereotypes having become even more negative, despite efforts to counteract these beliefs (Nelson 2017; Ng et al. 2015). The consequences of ageism are evident on many fronts, ranging from the immediate situational effects of age discrimination to the more distant impacts on well-being and longevity at population levels. Moreover, inculcating positive age attitudes at younger ages can shape positive attitudes and well-being at later ages (Levy 2022). A variety of factors have been implicated in ageism and its consequences including rising intergenerational tensions and generational biases directed toward younger adults (Francioli and North 2021). The neglect of age in academia, reflecting the historical, age-segregated model of higher education that builds inherent age barriers and fosters ageist practices, is also a contributing factor (Whitbourne and Montepare 2017). However, institutions of higher education offer teaching and learning environments that can combat ageist beliefs by implementing AFU principles and related practices. For example, advocating for expanding aging education, advancing awareness of the longevity dividend, and promoting intergenerational exchange help to tackle ageism through classroom efforts.

Evidence from studies in higher education using a variety of classroom strategies demonstrates the value of age-inclusive curricular and intergenerational practices. In particular, Levy's Positive Education about Aging and Contact Experiences (PEACE) model has argued that providing students with education about aging that includes facts on aging and positive models that dispel negative and inaccurate images of older adults, along with positive intergenerational experiences that are personal, cooperative, and promote equal status, and are central to reducing ageism (Levy 2018; Lytle and Levy 2019, 2022). Supporting the PEACE model and AFU principles, diverse studies have found that fostering students' knowledge about aging in college-level courses and providing them with opportunities for intergenerational exchange are effective in eliciting positive age attitudes. This includes courses with a specific aging focus (Hantman et al. 2013; Karasik et al. 2014; Wurtele and Maruyama 2013), specialized courses in the health professions (Gonzales et al. 2010), and non-aging-focused courses across the curriculum (Ermer et al. 2021; Lytle et al. 2020a, b; Montepare and Farah 2018). The evidence also includes experimental studies (Lytle et al. 2020a, b; Yamashita et al. 2018) and qualitative research (Augustin and Freshman 2016; Wagner and Luger 2021). Intergenerational contact beyond the classroom in community settings also offers valuable opportunities to counteract ageism (Andreoletti and Howard 2018; Leedahl et al. 2018; Stanley et al. 2019). If more campuses supported age-friendly educational strategies in the classroom and across the curriculum, progress would be made in challenging ageist stereotypes and altering age-biased behaviors.

It is also of interest to consider that traditional-age students may be especially receptive to disrupting ageist beliefs given their status as emerging adults, a stage during which many are open to exploring new ways of thinking, different life possibilities, and social relations (Arnett 2000). Intergenerational experiences can therefore be both developmentally and socially impactful in that they support solidarity between generations at a time when social trust and capital are eroding (Kaplan et al. 2017). Moreover, students may be especially sensitive to ageism given their experience of being stereotyped, profiled, and discriminated against for being young (Francioli and North 2021). Experiences with aging issues in families and career opportunities are also factors that set the stage for tackling ageism during the college years (Montepare and Pandolfi 2022).

AFU principles that advocate for community dialogue can also be seen as opportunities for disrupting ageism and reducing implicit age biases. The Reframing Aging Initiative (https://www.reframingaging.org/) provides an educational strategy designed to change the public discourse around aging through evidence-based modifications in the language used to communicate about aging and older adults (Reynolds 2020). Reframing involves adjusting how we talk about aging with respect to ideal versus real aging, individual versus collective control, attention to us versus them, and explanations that focus on fatalism versus mediating factors and possible solutions (https://www.reframingaging.org/). These adjustments in turn will impact how we think about aging. Recent research has found that reframing aging messages in this way can decrease implicit age bias—highlighting the value of incorporating research, education, and community collaborations on campuses to learn about and disseminate information about reframing communication strategies (Busso et al. 2019). Moreover, classroom settings and activities offer prime opportunities to engage students in discussions around the language of ageism so that they can recognize and rectify their own language-based age biases that fuel ageism as they prepare to move on to become community members (Gendron et al. 2016).

Final Comments

Efforts to advance age-friendly progress are mounting as the global population ages. With a firm understanding of the need for higher education to be more age-friendly, a growing network of committed AFU institutions, an emergent body of empirical research, and models of partnerships and possible eco-system connections, the future of age-friendly campuses is exciting and promising in this evolving environment. However, there is much to be done to break down structural barriers that hold institutions back from embracing age inclusivity, hone the AFU initiative, and coordinate efforts across age-friendly enterprises. As these challenges are met, age-friendly campuses will be integral to helping us all thrive in the new age-diverse world in which we live.

References

Age-Friendly University Global Network. n.d.. *Ten Principles of an Age-Friendly University*. Retrieved from https://www.afugn.org/principles

Andreoletti, C., and J.L. Howard. 2018. Bridging the Generation Gap: Intergenerational Service-learning Benefits Young and Old. *Gerontology & Geriatrics Education* 39 (1): 46–60. https://doi.org/10.1080/02701960.2016.1152266.

Arnett, J.J. 2000. Emerging Adulthood: A Theory of Development from the Late Teens Through the Twenties. *The American Psychologist* 55 (5): 469–480. https://doi.org/10.1037/0003-066X.55.5.469.

Augustin, F., and B. Freshman. 2016. The Effects of Service-learning on College Students' Attitudes toward Older Adults. *Gerontology & Geriatrics Education* 37 (2): 123–144. https://doi.org/10.1080/02701960.2015.1079705.

Busso, D.S., A. Volmert, and N. Kendall-Taylor. 2019. Reframing Aging: Effect of a Short-Term Framing Intervention on Implicit Measures of Age Bias. *The Journals of Gerontology: Series B* 74 (4): 559–564. https://doi.org/10.1093/geronb/gby080.

Cannon, M., R. Kerwood, M. Ramon, S.J. Rowley, and H. Rubio. 2021. Laying the Groundwork for an Age-Friendly University: A Multi-method Case Study. *Gerontology & Geriatrics Education* 44: 1–14. https://doi.org/10.1080/02701960.2021.1974016.

Chesser, S.A., M.M. Porter, R. Barclay, A.C. King, V.H. Menec, J. Ripat, K.M. Sibley, G.M. Sylvestre, and S.C. Webber. 2020. Exploring University Age-Friendliness Using Collaborative Citizen Science. *The Gerontologist* 60 (8): 1527–1537. https://doi.org/10.1093/geront/gnaa026.

Clark, P.G., and S.N. Leedahl. 2019. Becoming and Being an Age-Friendly University (AFU): Strategic Considerations and Practical Implications. *Gerontology & Geriatrics Education* 40 (2): 166–178. https://doi.org/10.1080/02701960.2019.1579714.

Corbie-Smith, G., S.B. Thomas, D.M.M. St, and George. 2002. Distrust, Race, and Research. *Archives of Internal Medicine* 162 (21): 2458. https://doi.org/10.1001/archinte.162.21.2458.

Coughlin, J. 2017. *The Longevity Economy: Unlocking the World's Fastest-Growing, Most Misunderstood Market*. Public Affairs Books.

Coyle, C.E., S.R. Gleason, and J.E. Mutchler. 2022. Spillover Benefits and Achieving Sustainability of Age-Friendly Communities. *Gerontologist* 62 (1): 29–35. https://doi.org/10.1093/geront/gnab060.

De Biasi, A., M. Wolfe, J. Carmody, T. Fulmer, and J. Auerbach. 2020. Creating an Age-Friendly Public Health System. *Innovation in Aging* 4 (1): 1–11. https://doi.org/10.1093/geroni/igz044.

DiSilvestro, F.R. 2013. Continuing Higher Education and Older Adults: A Growing Challenge and Golden Opportunity. *New Directions for Adult and Continuing Education* 140: 79–87. https://doi.org/10.1002/ace.20076.

Dugan, E., F. Porell, N.M. Silverstein, and C.M. Lee. 2022. Healthy Aging Data Reports: Measures of Community Health to Identify Disparities and Spur Age-Friendly Progress. *Gerontologist* 62 (1): e28–e38. https://doi.org/10.1093/geront/gnab111.

Eppler-Hattab, R., I. Meshoulam, and I. Doron. 2020. Conceptualizing Age-Friendliness in Workplaces: Proposing a New Multidimensional Model. *The Gerontologist* 60 (1): 12–21. https://doi.org/10.1093/geront/gny184.

Ermer, A.E., K. York, and K. Mauro. 2021. Addressing Ageism Using Intergenerational Performing Arts Interventions. *Gerontology & Geriatrics Education* 42 (3): 308–315. https://doi.org/10.1080/02701960.2020.1737046.

Filinson, R., and M. Raimondo. 2019. Promoting Age-Friendliness: One College's "Town and Gown" Approach to Fostering Community-based and Campus-wide Initiatives for Inclusiveness. *Gerontology & Geriatrics Education* 40 (3): 307–321. https://doi.org/10.1080/02701960.2019.1579715.

Francioli, S.P., and M.S. North. 2021. Youngism: The Content, Causes, and Consequences of Prejudices Toward Younger Adults. *Journal of Experimental Psychology: General* 150 (12): 2591–2612. https://doi.org/10.1037/xge0001064.

Fulmer, T., P. Patel, N. Levy, K. Mate, A. Berman, L. Pelton, J. Beard, A. Kalache, and J. Auerbach. 2020. Moving Toward a Global Age-Friendly Ecosystem. *Journal of the American Geriatrics Society* 68 (9): 1936–1940. https://doi.org/10.1111/jgs.16675.

Gendron, T.L., E.A. Welleford, J. Inker, and J.T. White. 2016. The Language of Ageism: Why We Need to Use Words Carefully. *The Gerontologist* 56 (6): 997–1006. https://doi.org/10.1093/geront/gnv066.

Gerontological Society of America. 2018. *Longevity Economics: Leveraging the Advantages of an Aging Society*. Retrieved from https://www.geron.org/programs-services/alliances-and-multi-stakeholder-collaborations/longevity-economics

Gonzales, E., N. Morrow-Howell, and P. Gilbert. 2010. Changing Medical Students' Attitudes Toward Older Adults. *Gerontology & Geriatrics Education* 31 (3): 220–234. https://doi.org/10.1080/02701960.2010.503128.

Grawe, N. 2018. *Demographics and the Demand for Higher Education*. Johns Hopkins University Press.

Gugliucci, M.R., and D. O'Neill. 2019. Health Professions Education: Advancing Geriatrics and Gerontology Competencies Through Age-Friendly University (AFU) Principles. *Gerontology & Geriatrics Education* 40 (2): 194–202. https://doi.org/10.1080/02701960.2019.1576658.

Hansen, R.J., C.A. Talmage, S.P. Thaxton, and R.C. Knopf. 2019. Barriers to Age-Friendly Universities (AFU): Lessons from Osher Lifelong Learning Institute Demographics and Perceptions. *Gerontology & Geriatrics Education* 40 (2): 221–243. https://doi.org/10.1080/02701960.2019.1572003.

Hantman, S., M.B. Oz, C. Gutman, and W. Criden. 2013. Bringing Older Adults into the Classroom: The Sharing Community Model. *Gerontology & Geriatrics Education* 34 (2): 135–149. https://doi.org/10.1080/02701960.2012.679372.

Hertzog, C., A.F. Kramer, R.S. Wilson, and U. Lindenberger. 2008. Enrichment Effects on Adult Cognitive Development: Can the Functional Capacity of Older Adults be Preserved and Enhanced? *Psychological Science in the Public Interest: A Journal of the American Psychological Society* 9 (1): 1–65. https://doi.org/10.1111/j.1539-6053.2009.01034.x.

June, A., and C. Andreoletti. 2023. Using an Age-Friendly University Lens to Explore Community Member Engagement During the Pandemic. *Gerontology & Geriatrics Education* 44 (1): 27–40. https://doi.org/10.1080/02701960.2021.2005039.

Kaplan, M., M. Sanchez, and J. Hoffman. 2017. *Intergenerational Pathways to a Sustainable Society*. Springer.

Karasik, R.J., R. Hamon, J. Writz, and A.M. Reddy. 2014. Two Thumbs Up: Using Popular Films in Introductory Aging Courses. *Gerontology & Geriatrics Education* 35 (1): 86–113. https://doi.org/10.1080/02701960.2012.749253.

Karasik, R.J., L. Donorfio, and P.A. Greenberg. 2022. *The Gerontology Field Placement: Internships and Practicums in Aging*. Springer.

Kehoe, B., F. Skelly, N. Moyna, M. Cantwell, L. Boran, L. Daly, A. McCarren, K. Dowd, C. Woods, N. McCaffrey, and L. Loughney. 2020. The Effect of Participating in Medex Wellness, a Community-Based Chronic Disease Exercise Rehabilitation Programme, on Physical, Clinical and Psychological Health: A Study Protocol for a Cohort Trial. *Contemporary Clinical Trials Communication* 18 (19): 100591. https://doi.org/10.1016/j.conctc.2020.100591.

Larkin, M.B., L. Mullane, and S.P. Robinson. 2007. *Framing New Terrain: Older Adults and Higher Education.* (No. 1). Washington DC: American Council on Education.

Leedahl, S.N., M.S. Brasher, E. Estus, B.M. Breck, C.B. Dennis, and S.C. Clark. 2018. Implementing an Interdisciplinary Intergenerational Program Using the Cyber Seniors® Reverse Mentoring Model Within Higher Education. *Gerontology & Geriatrics Education* 40 (1): 1–19. https://doi.org/10.1080/02701960.2018.1428574.

Lenehan, M.E., M.J. Summers, N.L. Saunders, J.J. Summers, D.D. Ward, K. Ritchie, and J.C. Vickers. 2016. Sending Your Grandparents to University Increases Cognitive Reserve: The Tasmanian Healthy Brain Project. *Neuropsychology* 30: 525–531. https://doi.org/10.1037/neu0000249.

Levy, S.R. 2018. Toward Reducing Ageism: PEACE (Positive Education about Aging and Contact Experiences) Model. *The Gerontologist* 58 (2): 226–232. https://doi.org/10.1093/geront/gnw116.

Levy, B. 2022. *Breaking the Age Code: How Your Beliefs About Aging Determine How Long and Well You Live*. Harper Collins.

Lim, J.S., M.-B. Park, C.H. O'Kelly, R.C. Knopf, and C.A. Talmage. 2022. A Tool for Developing Guidelines for Institutional Policy: A 60 Indicator Inventory for Assessing the Age-Friendliness of a University. *Educational Gerontology* 49 (3): 214–227. https://doi.org/10.1080/03601277.2022.2096326.

Lövdén, M., L. Fratiglioni, M.M. Glymour, U. Lindenberger, and E.M. Tucker-Drob. 2020. Education and Cognitive Functioning Across the Life Span. *Psychological Science in the Public Interest* 21 (1): 6–41. https://doi.org/10.1177/1529100620920576.

Luz, C., and R. Baldwin. 2019. Pursuing Age-Friendly University (AFU) Principles at a Major University: Lessons in Grassroots Organizing. *Gerontology & Geriatrics Education* 40 (3): 290–306. https://doi.org/10.1080/02701960.2019.1583224.

Lytle, A., and S.R. Levy. 2019. Reducing Ageism: Education about Aging and Extended Contact with Older Adults. *The Gerontologist* 59 (3): 580–588. https://doi.org/10.1093/geront/gnx177.

Lytle, A., and S. R. Levy. 2022. Reducing Ageism Toward Older Adults and Highlighting Older Adults as Contributors During the COVID-19 Pandemic. *Journal of Social Issues* 78 (4): 1066–1084. https://doi.org/10.1111/josi.12545.

Lytle, A., J. Macdonald, M. Apriceno, and S.R. Levy. 2020a. Reducing Ageism with Brief Videos About Aging Education, Ageism, and Intergenerational Contact. *The Gerontologist* 61 (7): 1164–1116. https://doi.org/10.1093/geront/gnaa167.

Lytle, A., N. Nowacek, and S.R. Levy. 2020b. Instapals: Reducing Ageism by Facilitating Intergenerational Contact and Providing Aging Education. *Gerontology & Geriatrics Education* 41 (3): 308–319. https://doi.org/10.1080/02701960.2020.1737047.

McGuire, S.L., D.A. Klein, and D. Couper. 2005. Aging Education: A National Imperative. *Educational Gerontology* 31: 443–460. https://doi.org/10.1080/03601270590928170.

Meyer, W. 2022. *Older Adults Embrace New Careers in Research. University of Colorado Anschutz Medical Campus.* Retrieved from https://news.cuanschutz.edu/cctsi/energetic-older-adults-embrace-new-careers-in-research

Montepare, J.M. 2019. Introduction to the Special Issue-Age-Friendly Universities (AFU): Principles, Practices, and Opportunities. *Gerontology & Geriatrics Education* 40 (2): 139–141. https://doi.org/10.1080/02701960.2019.1591848.

Montepare, J. M. 2021. *Benchmarking Age-Friendly University (AFU) Practices: Age-Friendly Inventory and Campus Climate Survey (ICCS) Study Insights* [Conference session]. Annual meeting of the Gerontological Society of America, Phoenix, AZ.

Montepare, J.M., and L.M. Brown. 2022. Age-Friendly Universities (AFU): Combating and Inoculating Against Ageism in a Pandemic and Beyond. *Journal of Social Issues* 78 (4): 1017–1037. https://doi.org/10.1111/josi.12541.

Montepare, J.M., and K.S. Farah. 2018. Talk of Ages: Using Intergenerational Classroom Modules to Engage Older and Younger Students Across the Curriculum. *Gerontology & Geriatrics Education* 39 (3): 385–394. https://doi.org/10.1080/02701960.2016.1269006.

Montepare, J.M., and G. Pandolfi. 2022. Students' Dementia Experience, Knowledge, and Concern: An Opportunity for Age-Friendly University (AFU) Programming. *Gerontology & Geriatrics Education* 43 (2): 163–172. https://doi.org/10.1080/02701960.2020.1793139.

Moos, R.H., and B.S. Moos. 1983. Adaptation and the Quality of Life in Work and Family Settings. *Journal of Community Psychology* 11 (2): 158–170. https://doi.org/10.1002/1520-6629(198304).

Morrow-Howell, N., E.F. Lawlor, E.S. Macias, E. Swinford, and J. Brandt. 2020. Making the Case for Age-Diverse Universities. *The Gerontologist* 60 (7): 1187–1193. https://doi.org/10.1093/geront/gnz181.

Morrow-Howell, N., N. Galucia, E. Swinford, and T. Meyer. 2022. Challenges and Opportunities of Age Diverse Universities: Perspectives from Admissions and Career Services. *Gerontology & Geriatrics Education*. https://doi.org/10.1080/02701960.2020.1864345.

Moye, J., M.J. Karel, K.E. Stamm, S.H. Qualls, D.L. Segal, Y.N. Tazeau, and D.A. DiGilio. 2019. Workforce Analysis of Psychological Practice with Older Adults: Growing Crisis Requires Urgent Action. *Training & Education in Professional Psychology* 13 (1): 46–55. https://doi.org/10.1037/tep0000206.

Neal, M.B., A.K. DeLaTorre, and P.C. Carder. 2014. Age-Friendly Portland: A University-City-Community Partnership. *Journal of Aging and Social Policy* 26 (1–2): 88–101. https://doi.org/10.1080/08959420.2014.854651.

Nelson, T., ed. 2017. *Ageism: Stereotyping and Prejudice Against Older Persons*. 2nd ed, 263–290. MIT Press.

Ng, R., H.G. Allore, M. Trentalange, J.K. Monin, and B.R. Levy. 2015. Increasing Negativity of Age Stereotypes across 200 Years: Evidence from a Database of 400 Million Words. *PLoS One* 10 (2): e0117086. https://doi.org/10.1371/journal.pone.0117086.

O'Kelly, C. 2015. Age-*Friendly University Annual Report*. Retrieved from https://www.dcu.ie/sites/default/files/agefriendly/afu_annual_report_complete.pdf

Park, D., J. Lodi-Smith, L. Drew, S. Haber, A. Hebrank, G.N. Bischof, and W. Aamodt. 2014. The Impact of Sustained Engagement on Cognitive Function in Older Adults: The Synapse Project. *Psychological Science* 25: 103–112. https://doi.org/10.1177/0956797613499592.

Pew Research Center. 2016. *Lifelong Learning and Technology*. Retrieved from https://www.pewresearch.org/internet/2016/03/22/lifelong-learning-and-technology/

Pritchard, A., J. Li, J. McChesney, and J. Bichsel. 2019. *The Challenges of an Aging Higher Ed Workforce*. Retrieved from https://www.cupahr.org/surveys/research-briefs/

Reynolds, L. 2020. The COVID-19 Pandemic Exposes Limited Understanding of Ageism. *Journal of Aging & Social Policy* 32 (4/5): 499–505. https://doi.org/10.1080/08959420.2020.1772003.

Richards, J. 2020. Assessment of the Current State of the 60-Year Curriculum and Research Agenda for the Future. In *The 60-Year Curriculum*, ed. C. Dede and J. Richards, 142–155. New York: Routledge.

Sánchez, M., and M. Kaplan. 2014. Intergenerational Learning in Higher Education: Making the Case for Multi-generational Classrooms. *Educational Gerontology* 40 (7): 473–485. https://doi.org/10.1080/03601277.2013.844039.

Schumacher, J., N. Brandt, B. Resnick, A. Nahabedian, M. Heavner, G. Netzer, L. Wilson, and R.E. Kheirbek. 2022. Merging an Age-Friendly University with An Age-Friendly Health Care System: Case Study Findings. *Innovation in Aging* 6 (Supplement 1): 568–569.

Silverstein, N., S.K. Whitbourne, L.M. Bowen, J.M. Montepare, C. Beaulieu, T. Jansen, and A. Prasad. 2021. Assessing Age Inclusivity in Higher Education: Introducing the Age-Friendly Inventory and Campus Climate Survey (ICCS). *The Gerontologist* 62 (1): e48–e61. https://doi.org/10.1093/geront/gnab090.

Simon, A., S. Masinda, and A. Zakrajsek. 2020. Age-Friendly University Environmental Scan: Exploring "Age-Friendliness" with Stakeholders at One Regional Comprehensive University. *Gerontology & Geriatrics Education*. https://doi.org/10.1080/02701960.2020.1783259.

Stanley, J.T., L.B. Morrison, B.A. Webster, J.R. Turner, and C.J. Richards. 2019. An Age-Friendly University (AFU) Assists with Technology Learning and Social Engagement Among Older Adults and Individuals with Developmental Disabilities. *Gerontology & Geriatrics Education* 40 (2): 261–275. https://doi.org/10.1080/02701960.2019.1572009.

Sánchez, M., and M. Kaplan. 2014. Intergenerational Learning in Higher Education: Making the Case for Multigenerational Classrooms. *Educational Gerontology 40*(7):473–485.https://doi.org/10.1080/03601277.2013.844039.

U.S. Census Bureau. 2020. *65 and Older Population Grows Rapidly as Baby Boomers Age*. Retrieved from https://www.census.gov/newsroom/press-releases/2020/65-older-population-grows.html

Van Horn, C.E., K. Krepcio, and M. Heidkamp. 2015. *Improving Education and Training for Older Workers [Research Report]*. Rutgers. Retrieved from https://www.heldrich.rutgers.edu/sites/default/files/2020-10/report-improving-education-training-older-workers-AARP-ppi.pdf

Wagner, L.S., and T.M. Luger. 2021. Generation to Generation: Effects of Intergenerational Interactions on Attitudes. *Educational Gerontology* 47 (1): 1–12. https://doi.org/10.1080/03601277.2020.1847392.

Whitbourne, S.K., and J.M. Montepare. 2017. What's Holding Us Back? Ageism in Higher Education. In *Ageism: Stereotyping and Prejudice Against Older Persons*, ed. T. Nelson, 2nd ed., 263–290. Cambridge: MIT Press.

Wurtele, S.K., and L. Maruyama. 2013. Changing Students' Stereotypes of Older Adults. *Teaching of Psychology* 40 (1): 59–61. https://doi.org/10.1177/0098628312465867.

Yamashita, T., S.J. Hahn, J.M. Kinney, and L.W. Poon. 2018. Impact of Life Stories on College Students' Positive and Negative Attitudes Toward Older Adults. *Gerontology & Geriatrics Education* 39 (3): 326–340. https://doi.org/10.1080/02701960.2017.1311884.

Chapter 5
Age-Friendly Health

Katarina Friberg-Felsted and Patricia M. D'Antonio

Age-friendly health is a critical component of the age-friendly ecosystem. Aging across the life course is as varied of an experience as humans are. Adults move through life into older adulthood under the effects of a variety of genetics, social determinants, and choices. While older adulthood is often a time of generativity, increased wisdom, and high satisfaction, older people are also exposed to and affected by ageism. Ageism is not only directly damaging to older people but also a costly bias to our communities and society. A variety of interventions have been researched to combat ageism, and many show promise. Fostering age-friendly health care is one solution to existing ageism. Ensuring that all elements of age-friendly health systems are evident in the care of all older people is highly recommended.

Ageism

Ageism has been defined in several ways. It is a stereotyping, prejudice, and/or discrimination directed at others related to aging, old/er age, older adults, older people, or aging processes; Robert Butler famously described it as another form of bigotry (Angus and Reeve 2006; Butler 1969; Hagestad and Uhlenberg 2006; Officer et al. 2016). While this discrimination is often common and even socially

K. Friberg-Felsted (✉)
Gerontology Interdisciplinary Program, College of Nursing, The University of Utah, Salt Lake City, UT, USA
e-mail: katarina.felsted@nurs.utah.edu

P. M. D'Antonio
Policy and Professional Affairs, Gerontological Society of America, Washington, DC, USA

National Center to Reframe Aging, Washington, DC, USA

V. Chang Greer, L. S. Edelman (eds.), *Age-Friendly Ecosystems*, SpringerBriefs in Public Health, https://doi.org/10.1007/978-3-031-68361-9_5

accepted, it is a significant risk to health and well-being (Allen 2016; Lamont et al. 2015; Wurm et al. 2017). Ageism is based on a variety of falsehoods and is a factor in major life events as well as in routine smaller ways.

Allen also notes that due to its wide acceptance, ageism may be under-accounted for, as a result of society's unawareness of it (Allen et al. 2022b). Hagestad also notes the complacency toward ageism (2006), and Weir notes that it is often not included in organizational equity, diversity, and inclusion (EDI) policies and documentation (2023). A well-defined concern regarding the stereotyping involved in ageism is that it perpetuates itself through categorization. In individual evaluation, people are much more likely to apply set stereotypes of the category they assign the individual rather than utilize the unique qualities of the individual (Montepare and Zebrowitz 2004). Hence, although an older person exhibits attributes that discredit ageist stereotypes, they will still be typecast within those stereotypical categories.

Everyday Ageism

"Everyday ageism" is recognized as the collection of messages and microaggressions that create negative associations with aging. Allen and colleagues define everyday ageism as "brief verbal, nonverbal, and environmental indignities that convey hostility, a lack of value, or narrow stereotypes of older adults" (2022a, 147). According to the National Poll on Healthy Aging (2020), ageism is extremely common, with 82 percent of adults aged 50–80 experiencing one or more forms of everyday ageism in their daily lives. The Poll also describes everyday ageist messages targeting two basic changes that tend to occur within aging: (1) health-related changes (such as difficulty with vision, hearing, or memory) as identity problems or character flaws and (2) changes in appearance or social behaviors as becoming less competent or desirable (2020).

Ageist microaggressions communicate to older people that they are considered other, not respected, or not valued (Allen et al. 2022a; Gietzen et al. 2023; Lewis 2023). Everyday interactions with strangers as well as family or friends are also vehicles for transmitting these microaggressions (Allen et al. 2022a) with friends, family, service providers, and strangers. Everyday ageism abounds in media and is found in the newly coined term "youngsplaining" (Comunello et al. 2022; Thayer and Skufca 2019). Chopik and Giasson noted that ageist attitudes are more explicit within younger age groups, while in older adults and older people, their presence is more implicit (2017). Everyday ageism was more strongly associated with lower economic status, rural areas, and higher media use. Everyday ageism is not always intentional and not always readily identified. According to Allen and colleagues, one characteristic of everyday ageism that causes it to be overlooked or discounted is that it may be perceived as humorous (black balloons on a 40th birthday), or considerate (speaking more slowly with assumed hearing impairment), or even flattering (Allen et al. 2022a).

A Threat to Physical and Mental Health

Everyday ageism is a form of chronic stress and increases the allostatic load in older adults (Allen et al. 2022a; Geronimus et al. 2006; Juster et al. 2010). Chronic stress is a risk factor for chronic disease, accelerated aging, and premature mortality (Allen 2016; Felsted 2020). It is noted that everyday ageism leads to poorer mental and physical health outcomes in older adults (Allen et al. 2022b; Hu et al. 2021; Lamont et al. 2015). This can be explained partially with Pearlin's stress process, which states that negative life events and chronic stressors may manifest as mental or physical symptoms, conditions, or diseases (Pearlin et al. 1981).

Internalized Ageism

Older adult individuals internalize this everyday ageism, and the pathways to negative health outcomes across a variety of physiological, psychological, and behavioral conditions are explained through stereotype embodiment theory, which notes that in response to continual exposure to ageist messages, older adults and older people absorb everyday ageism and internalize it (Allen 2016; Levy 2009). Scientific literature shows dozens of pathways between ageism and these conditions: chronic illnesses, depressive symptoms, cardiovascular syndromes, diabetes, higher levels of biomarkers of Alzheimer's disease, poor memory performance, and suicidal ideation (Allen et al. 2022a; Jackson et al. 2019; Levy et al. 2016). Underlining the directionality, Sargent-Cox and colleagues note that it is not negative changes in health that lead to ageism, but ageism that leads to negative changes in health (Sargent-Cox et al. 2012).

Ageism Within Employment

Older adults also face ageism within their careers, places of work, and employment. This appears as unemployment, underemployment, early forced retirement, and perceived employment scarcity (Abrams et al. 2016; Bender 2012; Ospina et al. 2019). Additionally, it affects hiring and promotion decisions and is a threat to career progression (Baska 2020; Lipnic, 2018; Surrportah, 2021; Wilson and Roscigno 2018).

Intersectionality with Ageism

Ageism must also be viewed through an intersectional lens. Prior research illuminates the overlapping and interdependence of other forms of discrimination, resulting in what is termed double jeopardy, triple jeopardy, or multiple jeopardy (Beale 2008; King 1988). These intersectionalities include gender, race, ableism/disability, and socioeconomic status, among others.

Gender

Women are often discriminated against in the context of ageism, with some literature showing this beginning in women's early 40s (Jaakson and Dedova 2023; Krekula et al. 2018). This discrimination is typically stronger than that directed toward older men (Calasanti et al. 2018; Chonody, 2015; Chrisler et al. 2016; Clarke and Korotchenko 2016). However, older men experience gendered ageism with relation to loss of physical performance as well as loss of career, even when voluntarily retiring (APA 2020; Kornadt et al. 2013). Within LGBTQ+ communities, lesbian, gay, and bisexual people experience more stress than do heterosexuals, and this stress leads to negative health outcomes (Meyer and Frost, 2013). Additionally, nearly half of LGBTQ+ older adults felt disrespected and/or invisible (Goldsen and Emlet 2021).

Disability/Ableism

Older adults are especially vulnerable to institutional ageism, which affects their abilities to seek and receive the types of accommodations offered to their younger counterparts (Jönson and Taghizadeh Larsson 2022; Chan et al. 2021). Disabled older adults are also more vulnerable to open shaming than able-bodied older adults (APA 2020; Larsson and Jönson 2018).

Race and Ethnicity

The additive effects of age and race result in poorer health for Hispanic and African American older adults. Another outcome of these combined biases is that African American and Hispanic older adults are left uninsured for longer parts of their lives, as compared to White older adults (Allen et al. 2019; Carreon and Noymer 2011; Kirby and Kaneda 2013). Takamura and colleagues also note that older adult Asian American women were the most victimized by acts of unprovoked violence against them during the coronavirus epidemic (2022).

Socioeconomic Status

One of the more insidious ageist beliefs is concentrated around older adults being perceived as not contributing to society. This is partially due to the unwillingness of society to recognize older adults' continued contributions (Abramset al. 2011; Martinez et al. 2011; Thanakwang and Isaramalai 2013). People aged 65 and older who are unhoused are even more vulnerable to ageist prejudices related to socioeconomic status (Canham et al. 2022).

Ageism Impacts Care Received by Older Adults

People who are older face institutional ageism, harmful both physically and mentally, in a myriad of settings (Abecassis et al. 2012; Briggs et al. 2012; Bryant et al. 2012; Buttigieg et al. 2018; Chang et al. 2020; Chrisler et al. 2016; Meisner 2012; Wurm et al. 2017; Wyman et al. 2018). Older adults are routinely excluded from clinical trials, even as the conditions, symptoms, and treatments are those that most directly affect them (Herrera et al. 2010; Nguyen et al. 2022). Regarding physical health, ageist attitudes affect the number of nurses, physicians, and healthcare providers who are trained and specialize in the care of older adults (Bodner et al., 2018; Higashi et al., 2012; Sonnega and Weir 2014). Regarding mental health, psychotherapists show bias against working with older patients, erroneously assume that depression is a normal part of aging, and make less favorable diagnoses and prognoses for older patients (APA 2020). According to Levy and colleagues, ageism's cost per year is $63 billion (Levy et al. 2020). Burnes and colleagues suggest that global health strategies need to consider ageism as a modifiable risk factor (2019).

Acting on Ageism and Health

Reducing ageism is key to improving human health, according to the World Health Organization (2015). They cite three reasons why ageism needs to be addressed: (1) human rights, (2) fostering sustainable development, and (3) imperative to adapt to shifts in the age structure.

The initial reason to dedicate resources to improve older adult health is the human right to the "highest attainable standard of health" (World Health Organization 2015, 14). This requires the establishment and adherence to a variety of policies, laws, and behaviors that, in turn, create the conditions that ensure this right for older people (Doron and Apter 2010; Kalache 2012). Baer and colleagues illustrate that this right to health includes availability, accessibility, and acceptability (2016).

The idea of fostering sustainable development entails that since older people will be an increasingly significant portion of the population, development needs to acknowledge the contributions that older adults make to society and ensure that they are included (World Health Organization 2015). Older people contribute both financially and socially to society, and policy changes need to consider their well-being for the larger well-being of society (Aboderin and Beard 2015; Ageing in the Twenty-first Century 2012; Bock et al. 2014; BoomAgers 2012; United Nations 2002).

Finally, it is imperative to adapt to shifts in the aging population that maximize older adult contributions while minimizing expenses associated with the aging of the population. As various models are utilized, it is critical to note whether they are providing proper information. For example, the dependency ratio model that compares the working population with the retired population, by comparing adults 64 and younger with adults 65 and older makes the ageist assumption that those older than 65 are retired. However, the US Bureau of Labor Statistics shows that 16.8 percent of adults 65 and over are still working (2023). Another example is referring to healthcare costs of older adults as the cost of older adults to society. Yet these figures must also be accompanied by tax revenue, economic spending, and tangible benefits collected from the same population (Cook 2011; World Population Prospects 2014; Wöss and Türk 2011).

The Role of Communication Strategies to Improve Understanding of Aging

Key to improving how the public understands aging is how communication occurs. The words society uses matter. Changing the way individuals speak, write, and portray older people will change attitudes about aging and ultimately advance the policies and programs that support us at every age and stage of life. Research from the National Center to Reframe Aging and its partner, the FrameWorks Institute, found that the public's perception of aging is decidedly negative and antithetical to how most older people feel and what experts in the field find to be true (Sweetland et al. 2017).

Furthermore, the research demonstrated that while the aging experts and advocates are providing messages that make perfect sense within the aging field, the public does not hear the messages in the way the experts intended. In the absence of knowledge, the public creates cultural models or mental shortcuts that help process information based on assumptions that come from past experiences or prior understandings. Because these cultural models are based on largely automatic assumptions, they can get in the way of engaged thinking about an issue. This has implications for those default assumptions that can obstruct people's ability to interpret the message as intended. Knowing what cultural models people have for thinking about aging issues and knowing which models are helpful or not helpful in steering people toward more productive ways of reasoning provide aging advocates with a strategic advantage.

In testing models, researchers have learned to position an aging society as an untapped resource by comparing aging to forward momentum, hence reframing the public's thinking by telling the story. The arc of the story includes why it matters (value), how it works (metaphor), and what solutions can be adopted (concrete solutions). Using a metaphor of building momentum provides people with new language for talking about aging—something quite different from the currently available cultural idioms (e.g., "fighting" or "battling" aging, the importance of "staying young"). These narratives were shown to effectively reduce ageism and promote more productive perceptions about aging. Research demonstrates that applying these framing strategies in communications can decrease implicit bias against older adults (Busso et al. 2019).

The key to providing an effective message is to avoid traps that have been long thought to be useful. Avoid messages that emphasize individual actions to drive aging outcomes, highlight aging as the process of decline, refer to older people as the "other," create crisis messaging about the aging population, or compare with other forms of discrimination. These themes promote unintended effects in the public's thinking about the message. More importantly, messages should create a context to help shape decisions and outcomes, highlighting the benefits of being inclusive, and show how interventions can change outcomes. Messages tell the solution story that includes the systems, supports, and concrete solutions to the issue (Lindland et al. 2015).

The Role of Age-Friendly Health

The built and social environment must continue to address the global issue of ageism. Ageist attitudes and procedures are steadily erased through research, policies, and practices that include older people in their own aging experience (Angus and Reeve 2006). Researchers note that optimism and positive self-perceptions of aging reduce ageism and increase longevity (Levy et al. 2002; Wurm and Benyamini 2014). A powerful preventative countermeasure to the deleterious effects of ageism is the concept and model of age-friendly health care. A precursor to Age-Friendly Health Systems is the World Health Organization's Age-Friendly Primary Health Care Centres Toolkit (World Health Organization 2008).

Age-Friendly Health Systems

Age-Friendly Health Systems is an initiative and cooperative effort between the John A. Hartford Foundation and the Institute for Healthcare Improvement (IHI) which have partnered with the American Hospital Association and the Catholic Health Association of the United States (Cacchione 2020; Fulmer 2019; Institute for Healthcare Improvement 2019). According to the Institute for Healthcare Improvement (2019), the three aims of Age-Friendly Health Systems are to follow an essential set of evidence-based practices, cause no harm, and align with what matters to the older adult and their family caregiver/s.

The 4 M Framework

The first and key M of the 4Ms framework is *What Matters* (see Fig. 5.1). This M indicates that age-friendly health should know and align care with each older adult's specific health outcomes, goals, and care preferences, including, but not limited to, end-of-life care, and across settings of care. This is the most basic tenet of

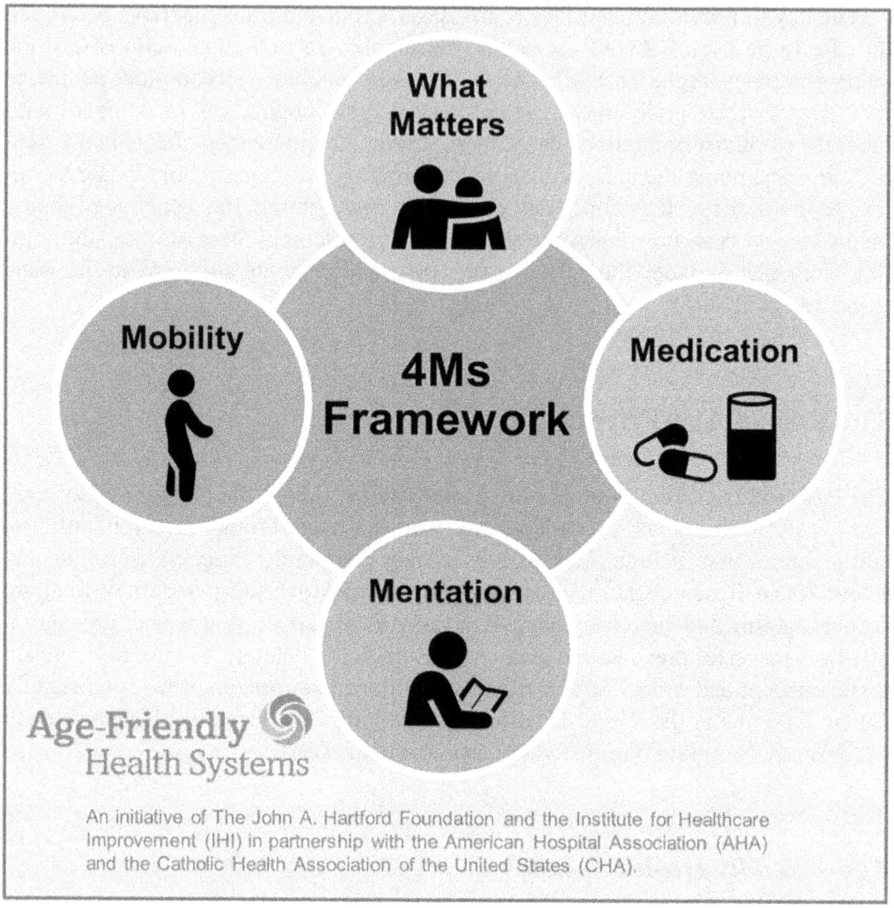

Fig. 5.1 4 M framework of an age-friendly health system. (Source: Reprinted with permission from Institute for Healthcare Improvement n.d. https://www.ihi.org/initiatives/age-friendly-health-systems

age-friendly care. Older people often receive care that is incongruent with their goals; often this care leads to poor health outcomes and actual unwanted care (Fulmer et al. 2023; Stuart et al. 2012). Instead, age-friendly health care combats ageism by respecting wisdom and self-actualization and valuing the experience, perspective, and judgment that accompany older age (Samuel 2022).

The second M of the 4 M framework is *Medication*. This indicates that if medication is necessary, age-friendly medication does not interfere with the other three Ms., What Matters, Mentation, and Mobility, across settings of care. The Age-friendly Health Systems framework focuses on reducing the harmful effects of medication use in older adults (IHI 2019). Fulmer and colleagues describe several medications that may be inappropriate for older people including highly anti-cholinergic medications, benzodiazepines, opioids, prescription and over-the-counter sedatives and sleep aids, and tricyclic antidepressants (2023). They recommend that the Age-friendly Health System complete a medication reconciliation and educate the older adult as well as their families and/or caregivers on appropriate medication use and/or discontinuation.

The third M of the 4 M framework, as mentioned above, is *Mentation*. This is a call to prevent, identify, treat, and manage dementia, depression, and delirium, across settings of care. An active approach within this M is the idea of screening early and often for delirium, as it responds well to acute care interventions, rather than viewing delirium as an early indicator of dementia (Fulmer et al. 2023). One successful model is the Hospital Elder Life Program, which "successfully prevents cognitive and functional decline in at-risk older patients" (Hshieh et al. 2018; Reuben et al. 2015, 1697). This preventative approach is at the heart of the Age-Friendly Health Systems 4 M framework. The Hospital Elder Life Program is found across many hospitals in the United States, the United Kingdom, Australia, Canada, and Taiwan (Rubin et al. 2011).

The fourth and final M of the 4 M framework is *Mobility*. This ensures that older adults move safely every day in order to maintain function and do What Matters. Mobility emphasizes the opposite of what care providers have focused on prior, the incidence and severity of falls; as such, this M again highlights ability instead of disability in older adults (Klein et al. 2023).

This framework addresses older adult health in a revolutionary way, by focusing on the health and well-being of older adults, rather than their diseases, functions, or chronic conditions (Fulmer et al. 2023). This focus encourages a reduction in ageist attitudes and approaches. While countries differ greatly in the type of health care and access they provide to their older adult population, the 4 M framework serves as a global guide.

Becoming Age-Friendly as a Health System

For those eager to join the Age-Friendly Health initiative, the IHI provides three avenues. The first is through Action Communities. Action Communities allow teams of all types to prepare to reliably practice age-friendly health. IHI also has pathways to two levels of Age-Friendly Health Systems Recognition, with guides for hospitals, emergency rooms, surgeries, ambulatory practices, care clinics, nursing homes, and multiple sites (Age-Friendly Health Systems, 2023). The second avenue Age-Friendly Health Systems provides is through Do-It-Yourself (DIY) Participation. This option is for entities who want to begin practicing age-friendly care and are motivated to begin immediately. The third option available from IHI is the scale-up accelerator, which provides scaled support to spread system-wide (Age-Friendly Health Systems 2023). Research shows that while most clinicians agree that older adults require different care than younger adults, and the majority discuss each of the 4Ms with their patients, less than 40% are asking What *M*atters and aligning the older adult's care plan with this information (Lesser et al. 2022). Continued education about and implementation of the 4Ms is needed to provide high-quality, patient-centered care for older people.

Embracing Age-Friendly as a Caregiver

The 4Ms (What Matters, Medication, Mentation, and Mobility) also serve as a guide for caregivers (Table 5.1). Caregivers are often the liaison between the healthcare system and the older adult, ensuring that the three aims of age-friendly health care are intact: the older adult care recipient receives the best care possible, they are unharmed, and they are satisfied with the care they receive (Emery-Tiburcio et al. 2021). The caregiver role is an important one with each M. Regarding What Matters,

Table 5.1 Healthcare professional resources and tools for assessing and acting on the 4Ms

4Ms	Resources	Link
What matters	VitalTalk	www.vitaltalk.org
	Patient priorities care	https://patientprioritiescare.org
	The conversation project	https://theconversationproject.org
Medication	Deprescribing.org: resources for patients and health care providers	https://deprescribing.org/resources
	2019 updated Ags beers criteria for potentially inappropriate medication use in older adults	https://pubmed.ncbi.nlm.nih.gov/30693946
Mentation	AGS CoCare: Help	www.americangeriatrics.org/programs/ags-cocarer-help
	Catch-on online modules	http://catch-on.org/hp-home/hp-education
Mobility	CDC: *Preventing falls: a guide to implementing effective community-based fall prevention programs*	www.cdc.gov/homeandrecreationalsafety/pdf/falls/fallpreventionguide-2015-a.pdf
	Johns Hopkins medicine: activity and mobility promotion	www.hopkinsmedicine.org/physical_medicine_rehabilitation/education_training/amp/toolkit.html
	Measures	Link
What matters	Patient priorities care: resources for clinicians and health systems	https://patientprioritiescare.org/resources/clinicians-and-health-systems
Medication	Stopp/Start toolkit supporting medication review	www.valeofyorkccg.nhs.uk/seecmsfile/?id=3035&inline=1
Mentation	Delirium screening UB-2 delirium screen CAM Nu-DESC	UB-2: www.nursing.psu.edu/wp-content/uploads/2019/03/UB-2-with-disclaimer-fick_Delirium-Pocket-Cand_052118.pdf CAM: http://eddelirium.org/delirium-assessment/cam Nu-DESC: https://deliriumnetwork.org/wp-content/uploads/2018/05/NuDESC.pdf
	Dementia screening Mini-Cog cognitive impairment screening SLUMS examination MoCA	Mini-Cog: https://mini-cog.com SLUMS: www.slu.edu/medicine/internal-medicine/geriatric-medicine/aging-successfully/pdfs/slums_form.pdf MoCA: www.mocatest.org

(continued)

Table 5.1 (continued)

	Depression screening PHQ-2 PHQ-9 GDS	PHQ-2: www.chpscc.org/_literature_243927/The_Patient_Health_Questionnaire_(PHQ-2) PHQ-9: www.phqscreeners.eom/images/sites/g/files/g10060481/f/201412/PHQ-9_English.pdf GDS: https://web.stanford.edu/~yesavage/GDS.html
Mobility	CDC timed up and go mobility assessment	www.cdc.gov/steadi/pdf/TUG_test-print.pdf
	Johns Hopkins highest level of mobility scale	www.hopkinsmedicine.org/physical_medicine_rehabilitation/_downloads/jh-hlm-faq.pdf
	Tinetti performance oriented mobility assessment	www.leadingagemn.org/assets/docs/Tinetti-Balance-Gait-POMA.pdf
	Barthel index of activities of daily living	www.sralab.org/rehabilitation-measures/barthel-index

Source: Reprinted from Emery-Tiburcio et al. (2021)
Key: *AGS* American geriatrics society, *CAM* confusion assessment method, *CDC* centers for disease control and prevention, *GDS* geriatric depression scale, *MoCA* montreal cognitive assessment, *Nu-DESC* nursing delirium screening scale, *PHQ-2* patient health questionnaire-2, *PHQ-9* patient health questionnaire-9, *SLUMS* Saint Louis University mental status, *START* screening tool to alert to right treatment, *STOPP* screening tool of older persons' prescriptions, *UB-2* 2-item ultra-brief

the caregiver can help inform the healthcare team about what matters for the patient/care recipient. Within Medications, the caregiver often plays the confirmatory role regarding what medications, and what dosages, the patient/care recipient is taking and is also in a unique situation to note any positive or adverse effects. With Mentation, the caregiver can serve as an advocate for the patient/care recipient as well as provide input on incidences that the patient/care recipient may be unclear about or have forgotten. Finally, with Mobility, the caregiver is an invaluable partner with the healthcare team to learn about safe movement for the patient/care recipient.

Conclusion

While aging is a natural part of human experience, and often comes with grace, wisdom, continued health, and societal engagement, the process itself faces harmful biases and stereotypes. This ageism is costly, damaging, and life-threatening that remains global. How we communicate about aging is key to improving the public's understanding about aging. Age-friendly health care, in the specific form of Age-friendly Health Systems, provides a framework for appropriate care of older adult patients as well as a framework to assist caregivers of older adults. The 4Ms, What Matters, Medication, Mentation, and Mobility, each serve as important tenets in the provision of age-friendly care. Age-Friendly Health Systems may serve to reduce ageism through their educational and humane care of older adults and older people, and this should be explored in future research.

References

Abecassis, M., N.D. Bridges, C.J. Clancy, et al. 2012. Solid-Organ Transplantation in Older Adults: Current Status and Future Research. *American Journal of Transplantation* 12 (10): 2608–2622. https://doi.org/10.1111/j.1600-6143.2012.04245.x.

Aboderin, I.A.G., and J.R. Beard. 2015. Older People's Health in Sub-Saharan Africa. *The Lancet* 385 (9968): E9–E11. https://doi.org/10.1016/S0140-6736(14)61602-0.

Abrams, D., P.S. Russell, M. Vauclair, and H.J. Swift. 2011. A Snapshot of Ageism in the UK and Across Europe. Technical Report. AgeUK. https://kar.kent.ac.uk/29735/

Abrams, D., H.J. Swift, and L. Drury. 2016. Old and Unemployable? How Age-Based Stereotypes Affect Willingness to Hire Job Candidates. *Journal of Social Issues* 72 (1): 105–121. https://doi.org/10.1111/josi.12158.

Age-Friendly Health Systems. 2023. Institute of Healthcare Improvement. https://www.ihi.org/initiatives/age-friendly-health-systems

Ageing in the Twenty-first Century: A Celebration and a Challenge. 2012. HelpAge International. New York, London: United Nations Population Fund. http://www.unfpa.org/sites/default/files/pub-pdf/Ageing%20report.pdf

Allen, J.O. 2016. Ageism as a Risk Factor for Chronic Disease. *The Gerontologist* 56 (4): 610–614. https://doi.org/10.1093/geront/gnu158.

Allen, J.O., D.C. Watkins, L. Chatters, A.T. Geronimus, and V. Johnson-Lawrence. 2019. Cortisol and Racial Health Disparities Affecting Black Men in Later Life: Evidence from MIDUS II. *American Journal of Men's Health* 13 (4): 1557988319870969. https://doi.org/10.1177/1557988319870969.

Allen, J.O., E. Solway, M. Kirch, D. Singer, J.T. Kullgren, and P.N. Malani. 2022a. The Everyday Ageism Scale: Development and Evaluation. *Journal of Aging and Health* 34 (2): 147–157. https://doi.org/10.1177/08982643211036131.

Allen, J.O., E. Solway, M. Kirch, D. Singer, J.T. Kullgren, V. Moïse, and P.N. Malani. 2022b. Experiences of Everyday Ageism and the Health of Older US Adults. *JAMA Network Open* 5 (6): e2217240.

American Psychological Association (APA). 2020. *APA Resolution on Ageism*.

Angus, J., and P. Reeve. 2006. Ageism: A Threat to "Aging Well" in the 21st Century. *Journal of Applied Gerontology* 25 (2): 137–152. https://doi.org/10.1177/0733464805285745.

Baer, B., A. Bhushan, H. Aout Taleb, J. Vasquez, and R. Thomas. 2016. The Right to Health of Older People. *The Gerontologist* 56 (Suppl 2): S206–S217. https://doi.org/10.1093/geront/gnw039.

Baska, M. 2020. Age Biggest Barrier to Career Progression, Survey Finds. *People Management*. https://www.peoplemanagement.co.uk/article/1742752/agebiggest-barrier-career-progression-survey-finds

Beale, F.M. 2008. Double Jeopardy: To be Black and Female. *Meridians* 8 (2): 166–176.

Bender, K.A. 2012. An Analysis of Well-Being in Retirement: The Role of Pensions, Health, and 'Voluntariness' of Retirement. *The Journal of Socio-Economics* 41 (4): 424–433. https://doi.org/10.1016/j.socec.2011.05.010.

Bock, J.-O., H. Matschinger, H. Brenner, B. Wild, W.E. Haefeli, R. Quinzler, K.-U. Saum, D. Heider, and H.-H. König. 2014. Inequalities in Out-of-Pocket Payments for Healthcare Services among Elderly Germans – Results of a Population-Based Cross-Sectional Study. *International Journal for Equity in Health* 13 (1): 3.

Bodner, E., Y. Palgi, and M.F. Wyman. 2018. Ageism in Mental Health Assessment and Treatment of Older Adults. In *Contemporary Perspectives on Ageism*, 241–262.

BoomAgers, N. 2012. *Introducing Boomers: Marketing's Most Valuable Generation*. New York: Nielsen.

Briggs, R., S. Robinson, and D. O'Neill. 2012. Ageism and Clinical Research. *Irish Medical Journal* 105 (9): 311–312.

Bryant, C.B., K. Bei, A. Gilson, H. Jackson Komiti, and F. Judd. 2012. The Relationship between Attitudes to Aging and Physical and Mental Health in Older Adults. *International Psychogeriatrics* 24 (10): 1674–1683.

Burnes, D., C. Sheppard, C.R. Henderson Jr., M. Wassel, R. Cope, C. Barber, and K. Pillemer. 2019. Interventions to Reduce Ageism Against Older Adults: A Systematic Review and Meta-Analysis. *American Journal of Public Health* 109 (8): e1–e9. https://doi.org/10.2105/AJPH.2019.305123.

Busso, D.S., A. Volmert, and N. Kendall-Taylor. 2019. Reframing Aging: Effect of a Short-Term Framing Intervention on Implicit Measures of Age Bias. *The Journals of Gerontology: Series B* 74 (4): 559–564.

Butler, R.N. 1969. Age-ism: Another Form of Bigotry. *Gerontologist* 9 (4): 243–246. https://doi.org/10.1093/geront/9.4_part_1.243.

Buttigieg, S.C., S. Ilinca, J.M. de Sao Jose, and A.T. Larsson. 2018. Researching Ageism in Health-Care and Long Term Care. In *Contemporary Perspectives on Ageism*, ed. L. Ayalon and C. Tesch-Römer, vol. 19, 493–515. Cham: Springer.

Cacchione, P.Z. 2020. Age-Friendly Health Systems: The 4Ms Framework. *Clinical Nursing Research* 29 (3): 139–140. https://doi.org/10.1177/1054773820906667.

Calasanti, T., N. King, I. Pietilä, and H. Ojala. 2018. Rationales for Anti-Aging Activities in Middle Age: Aging, Health, or Appearance? *The Gerontologist* 58 (2): 233–241.

Canham, S.L., J.N. Rose, R. Weldrick, E. Siantz, T. Casucci, and M.M. McFarland. 2022. Understanding Discrimination towards Persons Experiencing Homelessness: A Scoping Review Protocol. *BMJ Open* 12 (12): e066522.

Carreon, D., and A. Noymer. 2011. Health-Related Quality of Life in Older Adults: Testing the Double Jeopardy Hypothesis. *Journal of Aging Studies* 25 (4): 371–379. https://doi.org/10.1016/j.jaging.2011.01.004.

Chan, F., J.G. Dial, R. Schleser, B.T. McMahon, L.R. Shaw, M. Marmé, and C.S. Lam. 2021. An Ecological Approach to Vocational Evaluation. In *Work Worth Doing*, 115–133. Routledge.

Chang, E.-S., S. Kannoth, S. Levy, Y. Wang, J.E. Lee, and B.R. Levy. 2020. Global Reach of Ageism on Older Persons' Health: A Systematic Review. *PLoS One* 15 (1): e0220857.

Chonody, J.M. 2015. Addressing Ageism in Students: A Systematic Review of the Pedagogical Intervention Literature. *Educational Gerontology* 41 (12): 859–887.

Chopik, W.J., and H.L. Giasson. 2017. Age Differences in Explicit and Implicit Age Attitudes Across the Life Span. *The Gerontologist* 57 (Suppl. 2): S169–S177.

Chrisler, J.C., A. Barney, and B. Palatino. 2016. Ageism Can Be Hazardous to Women's Health: Ageism, Sexism, and Stereotypes of Older Women in the Healthcare System. *Journal of Social Issues* 72 (1): 86–104.

Clarke, L.H., and A. Korotchenko. 2016. 'I Know It Exists… but I Haven't Experienced It Personally': Older Canadian Men's Perceptions of Ageism as a Distant Social Problem. *Ageing & Society* 36 (8): 1757–1773.

Comunello, F., A. Rosales, S. Mulargia, F. Ieracitano, F. Belotti, and M. Fernández-Ardèvol. 2022. 'Youngsplaining' and Moralistic Judgements: Exploring Ageism Through the Lens of Digital 'Media Ideologies'. *Ageing and Society* 42 (4): 938–961.

Cook, J. 2011. The Socioeconomic Contribution of Older People in the UK. *Working with Older People* 15 (4): 141–146. https://doi.org/10.1108/13663661111191257.

Doron, I., and I. Apter. 2010. The Debate Around the Need for an International Convention on the Rights of Older Persons. *The Gerontologist* 50 (5): 586–593.

Emery-Tiburcio, E.E., L. Mack, M.C. Zonsius, E. Carbonell, and M. Newman. 2021. The 4Ms of an Age-Friendly Health System. *American Journal of Nursing* 121 (11): 44–49. https://doi.org/10.1097/01.NAJ.0000799016.07144.0d.

Felsted, K.F. 2020. Mindfulness, Stress, and Aging. *Clinics in Geriatric Medicine* 36 (4): 685–696. https://doi.org/10.1016/j.cger.2020.06.010.

Fulmer, T. 2019, February 11. Age-Friendly Health Ssystems Transform Care for Older Adults. Executive Insight in *Modern Healthcare*. John A. Hartford Foundation. https://www.johnahartford.org/images/uploads/reports/ModernHealthcareExecutiveInsight_TF_2.11.19.pdf

Fulmer, T., Berman, A., ,Lesiak, B., Alshabasy, S., and Levy, N. (2023). Age-Friendly Health Systems, in Gardiner, C. M., and Webb, E. O., Eds. The Age-Friendly Lens. DOI: https://doi.org/10.4324/9781003038658-6.

Geronimus, A.T., M. Hicken, D. Keene, and J. Bound. 2006. 'Weathering' and Age Patterns of Allostatic Load Scores Among Blacks and Whites in the United States. *American Journal of Public Health* 96 (5): 826–833.

Gietzen, L.J., H. Lewis, and J.A. Buchanan. 2023. Age-Related Microaggressions: A Descriptive Study. *The Gerontologist* 63 (5): 820–830.

Goldsen, K.F., and C. Emlet. 2021. Age Equity: A Framework for Addressing Ageism, Stigma, and Bias. *Innovation in Aging* 5 (S1): 431. https://doi.org/10.1093/geroni/igab046.1667.

Hagestad, G., and P. Uhlenberg. 2006. Should We Be Concerned About Age Segregation?: Some Theoretical and Empirical Explorations. *Research on Aging* 28 (6): 638–653. https://doi.org/10.1177/0164027506291872.

Herrera, A.P., S.A. Snipes, D.W. King, I. Torres-Vigil, D.S. Goldberg, and A.D. Weinberg. 2010. Disparate Inclusion of Older Adults in Clinical Trials: Priorities and Opportunities for Policy and Practice Change. *American Journal of Public Health* 100 (suppl 1): S105–S112.

Higashi, R.T., A.A. Tillack, M. Steinman, M. Harper, and C.B. Johnston. 2012. Elder Care as 'Frustrating' and 'Boring': Understanding the Persistence of Negative Attitudes toward Older Patients Among Physicians-in-Training. *Journal of Aging Studies* 26 (4): 476–483.

Hshieh, T.T., T. Yang, S.L. Gartaganis, J. Yue, and S.K. Inouye. 2018. Hospital Elder Life Program: Systematic Review and Meta-analysis of Effectiveness. *The American Journal of Geriatric Psychiatry* 26 (10): 1015–1033. https://doi.org/10.1016/j.jagp.2018.06.007.

Hu, R.X., M.S. Luo, A. Zhang, and L.W. Li. 2021. Associations of Ageism and Health: A Systematic Review of Quantitative Observational Studies. *Research on Aging* 43 (7–8): 311–322.

Institute for Healthcare Improvement. 2019. *Age-Friendly Health Systems: Guide to Using the 4Ms in the Care of Older Adults*.

———. n.d. *Age-Friendly Health Systems*. https://www.ihi.org/initiatives/age-friendly-health-systems

Jaakson, K., and M. Dedova. 2023. Do (Gendered) Ageism and Ethnic Minorities Explain Workplace Bullying? *International Journal of Manpower* 44 (9): 199–215.

Jackson, S.E., R.A. Hackett, and A. Steptoe. 2019. Associations Between Age Discrimination and Health and Wellbeing: Cross-Sectional and Prospective Analysis of the English Longitudinal Study of Ageing. *The Lancet Public Health* 4 (4): e200–e208. https://doi.org/10.1016/S2468-2667(19)30035-0.

Jönson, H., and A. Taghizadeh Larsson. 2022. Ableism and Ageism. In *Encyclopedia of Gerontology and Population Aging*, 4–9. Cham: Springer International Publishing.

Juster, R.-P., B.S. McEwen, and S.J. Lupien. 2010. Allostatic Load Biomarkers of Chronic Stress and Impact on Health and Cognition. *Neuroscience and Biobehavioral Reviews* 35 (1): 2–16.

Kalache, A. 2012. Human Rights in Older Age. In *Global Population Ageing: Peril or Promise?* ed. J.S. Beard, D.E. Bloom, L.P. Fried, P. Hogan, A. Kalache, et al., 89–92. Geneva: World Economic Forum.

King, Deborah K. 1988. Multiple Jeopardy, Multiple Consciousness: The Context of a Black Feminist Ideology. *Signs* 14 (1): 42–47. https://doi.org/10.1086/494491.

Kirby, J.B., and T. Kaneda. 2013. 'Double Jeopardy' Measure Suggests Blacks and Hispanics Face More Severe Disparities than Previously Indicated. *Health Affairs* 32 (10): 1766–1772. https://doi.org/10.1377/hlthaff.2013.0434.

Klein, S., R. Brondeel, B. Chaix, O. Klein, B. Thierry, Y. Kestens, P. Gerber, and C. Perchoux. 2023. What Triggers Selective Daily Mobility Among Older Adults? A Study Comparing Trip and Environmental Characteristics Between Observed Path and Shortest Path. *Health & Place* 79: 102730. https://doi.org/10.1016/j.healthplace.2021.102730.

Kornadt, A.E., P. Voss, and K. Rothermund. 2013. Multiple Standards of Aging: Gender-Specific Age Stereotypes in Different Life Domains. *European Journal of Ageing* 10: 335–344.

Krekula, C., P. Nikander, and M. Wilińska. 2018. Multiple Marginalizations Based on Age: Gendered Ageism and Beyond. *International Perspectives on Aging* 19: 33–50.

Kydd, A., and A. Fleming. 2015. Ageism and Age Discrimination in Health Care: Fact or Fiction: A Narrative Review of the Literature. *Maturitas* 81 (4): 432–438. https://doi.org/10.1016/j.maturitas.2015.05.002.

Lamont, R.A., H.J. Swift, and D. Abrams. 2015. A Review and Meta-analysis of Age-based Stereotype Threat: Negative Stereotypes, not Facts, Do the Damage. *Psychology and Aging* 30 (1): 180–193.

Larsson, A.T., and H. Jönson. 2018. Ageism and the Rights of Older People. In *Contemporary Perspectives on Ageism*, ed. L. Ayalon and C. Tesch-Römer, 369–382. Cham: Springer. https://doi.org/10.1007/978-3-319-73820-8_22.

Lesser, S., S. Zakharkin, C. Louie, M.R. Escobedo, J. Whyte, and T. Fulmer. 2022. Clinician Knowledge and Behaviors Related to the 4Ms Framework of Age-Friendly Health Systems. *Journal of the American Geriatrics Society* 70 (3): 789–800. https://doi.org/10.1111/jgs.17571.

Levy, B. 2009. Stereotype Embodiment: A Psychosocial Approach to Aging. *Current Directions in Psychological Science* 18 (6): 332–336. https://doi.org/10.1111/j.1467-8721.2009.01662.x.

Levy, B.R., M.D. Slade, S.R. Kunkel, and S.V. Kasl. 2002. Longevity Increased by Positive Self-perceptions of Aging. *Journal of Personality and Social Psychology* 83 (2): 261–270.

Levy, B.R., L. Ferrucci, A.B. Zonderman, M.D. Slade, J. Troncoso, and S.M. Resnick. 2016. A Culture-Brain Link: Negative Age Stereotypes Predict Alzheimer's Disease Biomarkers. *Psychology and Aging* 31 (1): 82–88. https://doi.org/10.1037/pag0000062.

Levy, B.R., M.D. Slade, E. Chang, S. Kannoth, and S.Y. Wang. 2020. Ageism Amplifies Cost and Prevalence of Health Conditions. *The Gerontologist* 60 (1): 174–181. https://doi.org/10.1093/geront/gny131.

Lewis, H.M. 2023. *Age-Related Microaggressions: A Follow-Up Descriptive Study*. Doctoral dissertation. Minnesota State University, Mankato.

Lindland, E., M. Fond, A. Haydon, and N. Kendall-Taylor. 2015. *Gauging Aging: Mapping the Gaps between Expert and Public Understandings of Aging in America*. Vol. 1, 211. Washington: FrameWorks Insitute.

Lipnic, V.A. 2018. *The State of Age Discrimination and Older Workers in the US 50 Years After the Age Discrimination in Employment Act (ADEA)*. Washington: US Equal Employment Opportunity Commission.

Martinez, I.L., D. Crooks, K.S. Kim, and E. Tanner. 2011. Invisible Civic Engagement Among Older Adults: Valuing the Contributions of Informal Volunteering. *Journal of Cross-Cultural Gerontology* 26: 23–37.

Meisner, B.A. 2012. A Meta-Analysis of Positive and Negative Age Stereotype Priming Effects on Behavior Among Older Adults. *Journals of Gerontology. Series B, Psychological Sciences and Social Sciences* 67 (1): 13–17.

Meyer, I.H., and D.M. Frost. 2013. Minority Stress and the Health of Sexual Minorities. In *Handbook of Psychology and Sexual Orientation*, ed. C.J. Patterson and A.R. D'Augelli, 252–266. Oxford University Press.

Montepare, J.M., and L.A. Zebrowitz. 2004. A Social-Developmental View of Ageism. In *Ageism: Stereotyping and Prejudice against Older Persons*, ed. T.D. Nielson. MIT Press. https://doi.org/10.7551/mitpress/1157.001.0001.

National Poll on Healthy Aging. 2020. *Everyday Ageism and Health*. https://www.healthyagingpoll.org/reports-more/report/everyday-ageism-and-health

Nguyen, D., G. Mika, and A. Ninh. 2022. Age-Based Exclusions in Clinical Trials: A Review and New Perspectives. *Contemporary Clinical Trials* 114: 106683.

Officer, A., M.L. Schneiders, D. Wu, P. Nash, J.A. Thiyagarajan, and J.R. Beard. 2016. Valuing Older People: Time for a Global Campaign to Combat Ageism. *Bulletin of the World Health Organization* 94 (10): 710–710A. https://doi.org/10.2471/BLT.16.184960.

Ospina, J.H., J.N. Cleveland, and A.M. Gibbons. 2019. The Relationship of Employment Scarcity and Perceived Threat with Ageist and Sexist Attitudes. *Work, Aging and Retirement* 5 (3): 215–235. https://doi.org/10.1093/workar/waz003.

Pearlin, L.I., E.G. Menaghan, M.A. Lieberman, and J.T. Mullan. 1981. The Stress Process. *Journal of Health and Social Behavior* 2 (4): 337–356.

Reuben, D.B., S.K. Inouye, S.T. Bogardus Jr., D.I. Baker, L. Leo-Summers, and L.M. Cooney Jr. 2015. The Hospital Elder Life Program: A Model of Care to Prevent Cognitive and Functional Decline in Older Hospitalized Patients. *Journal of the American Geriatrics Society* 48 (12): 1697–1706. https://doi.org/10.1111/j.1532-5415.2000.tb03885.x.

Rubin, F.H., K. Neal, K. Fenlon, S. Hassan, and S.K. Inouye. 2011. Sustainability and Scalability of the Hospital Elder Life Program at a Community Hospital. *Journal of the American Geriatrics Society* 59 (2): 359–365.

Samuel, L.R. 2022. *Age Friendly: Ending Ageism in America*. Routledge.

São José, J.M., C.A. Amado, S. Ilinca, S.C. Buttigieg, and Larsson A. Taghizadeh. 2019. Ageism in Health Care: A Systematic Review of Operational Definitions and Inductive Conceptualizations. *The Gerontologist* 59 (1): e98–e108.

Sargent-Cox, K.A., K.J. Anstey, and M.A. Luszcz. 2012. The Relationship Between Change in Self-Perceptions of Aging and Physical Functioning in Older Adults. *Psychology and Aging* 27 (3): 750.

Sonnega, A., and D.R. Weir. 2014. The Health and Retirement Study: A Public Data Resource for Research on Aging. *Open Health Data* 2: e7. https://doi.org/10.5334/ohd.am.

Stuart, B., K. Nguyen, and B. Gornet. 2012. System-Integrated Program Coordinates Care for People with Advanced Illness, Leading to Greater Use of Hospice Services, Lower Utilization and Costs, and High Satisfaction. In *AHRQ Innovations Exchange: Innovations and Tools to Improve Quality and Reduce Disparities*, 24.

Surpportah. 2021, October 18. *Construction and Recruitment Companies Penalised for Age Discrimination*. Retrieved from Human Rights Claims https://humanrightsclaims.com.au/construction-and-recruitment-penalised/

Sweetland, J., A. Volmert, and M. O'Neil. 2017. *Finding the Frame: An Empirical Approach to Reframing Aging and Ageism*. Washington: FrameWorks Institute.

Takamura, J.C., C. Browne, R. Jeung, A.J. Yellow Horse, D. Kwok, and D. Howard. 2022. Asian American Elders: Caught in the Crosshairs of a Syndemic of Racism, Misogyny, and Ageism During Coronavirus Disease 2019. *Public Policy and Aging Report* 32 (3): 87–93.

Thanakwang, K., and S.A. Isaramalai. 2013. Productive Engagement in Older Adults: A Concept Analysis. *Nursing & Health Sciences* 15 (1): 124–130. https://doi.org/10.1111/nhs.12015.

Thayer, C., and L. Skufca. 2019. *Media Image Landscape: Age Representation in Online Images*. Washington: AARP Research. https://doi.org/10.26419/res.00339.001.

U.S. Bureau of Labor Statistics. 2023. *Civilian Labor Force Participation Rate by Age, Sex, Race, and Ethnicity*. United States Department of Labor.

United Nations. 2002. *Political Declaration and Madrid International Plan of Action on Ageing*. Second World Assembly of Aging.

Weir, K. 2023. Ageism Is One of the Last Socially Acceptable Prejudices. Psychologists Are Working to Change That. *Monitor on Psychology* 54(2), American Psychological Association. Retrieved from https://www.apa.org/monitor/2023/03/cover-new-concept-of-aging

Wilson, G., and V.J. Roscigno. 2018. Race, Ageism and the Slide from Privileged Occupations. *Social Science Research* 69: 52–64.

World Economic Forum Global Agenda Council on Ageing Society. 2012.

World Health Organization. 2008. *Age-Friendly Primary Health Care Centres Toolkit*. World Health Organization. http://www.ncbi.nlm.nih.gov/books/NBK310500/

———. 2015, September 30. *World Report on Ageing and Health*. Available at https://www.who.int/publications/i/item/9789241565042

World Population Prospects: The 2012 Revision. 2014. *Methodology of the United Nations Population Estimates and Projections*. New York: United Nations Department of Economic and Social Affairs, Population Division.

Wöss, J., and E. Türk. 2011. *Dependency Ratios and Demographic Change. The Labour Market as a Key Element. ETUI Policy Brief*. Brussels: European Trade Union Institute.

Wurm, S., and Y. Benyamini. 2014. Optimism Buffers the Detrimental Effect of Negative Self-perceptions of Ageing on Physical and Mental Health. *Psychology & Health* 29 (7): 832–848. https://doi.org/10.1080/08870446.2014.891737.

Wurm, S., M. Diehl, A.E. Kornadt, G.J. Westerhof, and H.W. Wahl. 2017. How Do Views on Aging Affect Health Outcomes in Adulthood and Late Life? Explanations for an Established Connection. *Developmental Review* 46: 27–43. https://doi.org/10.1016/j.dr.2017.08.002.

Wyman, M.F., S. Shiovitz-Ezra, and J. Bengel. 2018. Ageism in the Health Care System: Providers, Patients, and Systems. In *Contemporary Perspectives on Ageism*, ed. L. Ayalon and C. Tesch-Römer, 193–212. Cham: Springer.

Chapter 6
Age-Friendly Voices in the Pursuit of an Age-Friendly Ecosystem

Sarah L. Canham and Timothy W. Farrell

Given the global aging of the population, there is a significant need to understand the facilitators and barriers to age-friendly neighborhoods, health systems, and campuses. To advance initiatives across the age-friendly ecosystem, we need to involve multiple stakeholders (Fulmer et al. 2020). In addition, given the heterogeneity in regional needs, local voices must be engaged in the development, implementation, and sustainment of age-friendly neighborhoods, health systems, and campuses. As there is no one way to be age-friendly, it is important to tailor initiatives to the uniqueness of each physical and social setting. Age-friendly concepts and principles are not intended to be mandates, but rather guiding principles to inform a holistic approach across places and sectors.

In regions attempting to achieve age-friendliness across diverse sectors, areas of overlap and synergy should be identified so that efforts complement and support shared goals rather than compete and complicate. To this end, this chapter describes recommendations for key stakeholders in the Intermountain West region of the United States to include in the development, implementation, and sustaining of age-friendly initiatives with the hope of informing efforts in other regions. The Intermountain West includes states in the western United States between the Rockies, Sierras, and Cascades, including Utah, Nevada, Idaho, as well as portions of Arizona, California, Colorado, Montana, New Mexico, Texas, Washington, and Wyoming (Burow et al. 2019). Relative to urban coastal regions, economies in the

S. L. Canham (✉)
College of Social Work, University Health Interprofessional Education Program, Healthy Aging and Resilient Places Lab, The University of Utah, Salt Lake City, UT, USA
e-mail: sarah.canham@utah.edu

T. W. Farrell
Division of Geriatrics, Spencer Fox Eccles School of Medicine, VA SLC Geriatric Research, Education, and Clinical Center, University of Utah Academy of Health Science Educators, The University of Utah, Salt Lake City, UT, USA

V. Chang Greer, L. S. Edelman (eds.), *Age-Friendly Ecosystems*, SpringerBriefs in Public Health, https://doi.org/10.1007/978-3-031-68361-9_6

Intermountain West are reliant on the amenities and resources of the natural environment, and there is a significant amount of public land managed by governmental agencies. In addition, the topography of the Intermountain West includes substantial open and rural spaces and mountainous terrain with large elevation differentials (Burow et al. 2019).

In this chapter, we describe lessons from a World Café workshop hosted during a 2-day virtual symposium that was undertaken in Fall 2022. World Café workshops offer opportunities for critical dialogue and cross-pollination of ideas between groups of individuals who have similar interests and expertise (Brown et al. 2009). In this instance, a 1.5-hour World Café session was held during a virtual symposium to collect data, share knowledge, and foster collaborative learning between participants (Fouché and Light 2011). Workshop participants included university faculty and students, community-based service providers, clinicians, and state employees in health and human services. Participants were asked about their perceptions of facilitators, barriers, priorities, innovations, and key stakeholders related to age-friendly neighborhoods, health systems, and campuses in the Intermountain West. Using the breakout room feature on Zoom, we divided participants into six rooms, and six discussion facilitators were assigned to one of three topics: (1) age-friendly neighborhoods, (2) age-friendly health systems, or (3) age-friendly campuses. Two facilitators were assigned to each age-friendly topic and navigated into and out of three different breakout rooms (facilitating discussions for 20 min in each), while participants remained in the same breakout room for the duration of the workshop.

In the following sections, we outline what we learned from participants about who the key stakeholders are—or should be—for creating age-friendly neighborhoods, health systems, and campuses in the Intermountain West and discuss areas of overlap across the different sectors. We hope this will offer insight into where synergies can be leveraged to advance age-friendly initiatives in other regions. Since age-friendly initiatives are inherently specific to their sociocultural contexts, knowing the narratives of age-friendly communities and stakeholders is important to empowering awareness, discussion, and collaboration. Moreover, critical reflection on who is or is not at the table is key to advancing commitments to diversity, equity, and inclusion within age-friendly work. Failure to understand whose voices are or are not at age-friendly planning tables may lead to inefficiencies or cross-sector competition for scarce resources. Alternatively, finding mechanisms for resource sharing, collaboration, and partnership may amplify and strengthen efforts. This idea is reflected by one workshop participant who stated:

> I would add the importance of collaborative efforts. Today I heard a couple of people mention all the amazing work that happens in silos and how to bring it all [together]. And that's really the concept of this age-friendly ecosystem and that's really great. But how do we build a network to really make that the norm?

Workshop participants suggested that the key stakeholder groups within the age-friendly ecosystem (see Fig. 6.1) include: (1) local age-friendly champion(s); (2) state and local policymakers and legislators; (3) healthcare departments and clinicians; (4) university leadership, faculty, and students; (5) businesses, religious

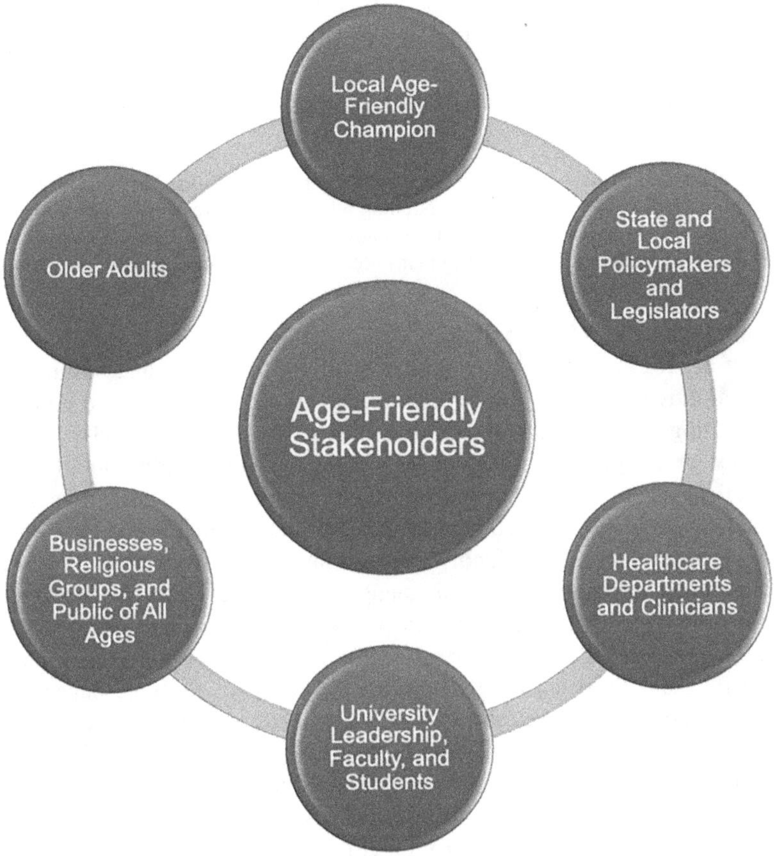

Fig. 6.1 Age-friendly stakeholders

groups, and the general public of all ages; and (6) older adults. These stakeholder groups have also been identified in the age-friendly literature (Fulmer et al. 2020), offering support for workshop participants' ideas on how to advance age-friendly initiatives in the Intermountain West.

Local Age-Friendly Champion(s)

Bringing in examples of how other communities have been successful in implementing and sustaining age-friendly initiatives, Portland, Oregon, was identified by one participant as a city that had "a dedicated champion to spearhead the effort" (see also Neal et al. 2014). Participants suggested that the qualifications for this age-friendly champion include being a well-respected and well-connected community leader in geriatrics or education, including being well connected with policymakers.

Successful age-friendly champions were described as having a vision and carrying this vision forward to obtain Age-Friendly City or Age-Friendly Health System designations. Though a single individual was not identified within the Intermountain West, the Utah Commission on Aging and AARP Utah were highlighted as local champion organizations:

> I think [the Commission on Aging is] one of our biggest facilitators. They convene across all sectors. . . . Such an amazing job of building relationships across silos, which is one of the reasons why I think we have symposiums now like this and we're having these discussions across so many disciplines and so many areas. So, I think that's a major facilitator for us here in the Intermountain West.

Community champions have been previously highlighted (Menec and Brown 2022; Russell et al. 2022) as a critical component to implementing and sustaining age-friendly initiatives given the leadership needed to organize and form committees, submit funding proposals, and move ideas into action. While some challenges with community champions have been identified, such as volunteer burnout or competing priorities, successes are increased through collaborations and partnerships that distribute the workload (Russell et al. 2022). As an example offered by World Café workshop participants, Age-Friendly Portland has been described as a "university-city-community collaborative" and inaugural member of the World Health Organization's (WHO) Global Network of Age-Friendly Cities (Neal et al. 2014, 2015). In this instance, the university researchers within the Institute on Aging (IOA) at Portland State University developed a series of resource papers for city planners and conducted research to identify the needs and capacity for Portland to be an age-friendly city (Neal et al. 2014). The IOA served as the coordinating organization by eliciting broad stakeholder input and translating data to policymakers (Neal et al. 2015). The Age-Friendly Portland Advisory Council, which included public, private, university, and nonprofit members, developed an action plan, monitored progress, and informed research. This work led to the formation of strong coalitions with shared goals and plans between university researchers, local city and government agency staff, and special interest groups (Neal et al. 2014).

State and Local Policymakers and Legislators

Across age-friendly neighborhoods, campuses, and health systems, state and local policymakers and legislators were identified by workshop participants as key stakeholders in the implementation and continuation of age-friendly initiatives. Initiating and sustaining age-friendly initiatives could be done, as suggested by one participant, "[By] our government leaders, for sure. With that messaging and prioritizing—it could be a prioritizing of funds, but also just getting the information out there, making it a priority, verbalizing them into priority." Participants suggested that government funding is key to the provision of agency resources and staff, and that buy-in from elected officials is integral to advancing initiatives. Moreover, policymakers were portrayed as having the power to make a structure that is less about financial gain and more about outcomes. While participants suggested that legislators who have had exposure to older adults and persons with disabilities are likely to be among the best advocates, as one participant stated, "If they are smart, they will advocate for aging because all of them are getting old." As exemplified by the Age-Friendly Portland efforts (Neal et al. 2014, 2015), offering relevant data, including demographic projections, to policymakers can serve as a powerful mechanism by which to engage and get buy-in from these decision-makers. Recommended strategies for sharing information with policymakers include condensing research evidence into brief and easy communications, including op-eds or policy briefs (Avey and Desch 2014). In addition, as elected officials need to be responsive to their constituents, there may be localized mechanisms by which to engage policymakers in community-based forums (Jackson-Elmoore 2005), including developing opportunities to meet older adults and age-friendly champions.

Workshop participants noted that challenges to engaging policymakers and legislators in age-friendly initiatives included the limited recognition that they are aging and may 1 day need home care, the lack of age-based retirement mandates for government decision-makers, and the high costs of Medicare, Medicaid, and other social entitlement programs. Embedded within these ideas are the ageist assumptions held by some that older adults may not be worth the higher costs of care they require (Farrell et al. 2022; Hamel et al. 2020).

Exemplars for including community leaders in age-friendly initiatives were shared by workshop participants. A participant who had attended a Dublin City University conference described how "mayors and council people. . .weren't just there to give support; they knew what was going on and they were integrated in the initiatives." In 2017, Governor Charles D. Baker of Massachusetts signed Executive Order 576 establishing a cross-sector *Council to Address Aging* inclusive of business, academic, health care, municipal, technology, advocacy, and community leaders (Office of the Governor 2019), which workshop participants thought gave credibility and validity to age-friendly issues. In the Intermountain West, there was appreciation for local policymakers who were described by one participant: "Our city and county mayors have been a little bit more public facing than in the past. . .support and [being able to] interact with has been great." Conversely, another participant felt that state legislators who are real estate developers have "some pretty defined ideas of what Utah ought to be," which hinders rezoning for the development of accessory dwelling units or other small housing types, which would support older residents to age in affordable locations.

Healthcare Departments and Clinicians

While participants in the age-friendly health systems breakout rooms had focused discussions on healthcare stakeholders, ideas about the roles of public health departments and clinicians were discussed across the ecosystem. In Utah, there are two primary health systems, University of Utah Health, an academic health sciences center, and Intermountain Health, a nonacademic organization with a larger market share. For one participant, there was hope for more system-level collaboration: "One of the things that would be interesting to me is how do they interact better? I think there's a lot of barriers in between these two very wonderful systems [e.g., communication]. . .but I see those large healthcare corporations as being key stakeholders." Primarily familiar with the University of Utah Health system, another participant described progress in getting an age-friendly designation, which is not a designation held by Intermountain Health.

> Well, being from the University of Utah, I can say that the University of Utah, as the Academic Health Sciences Center along the Wasatch Front, is very committed to being an Age-Friendly Health System. So, we have that process in place. And we heard yesterday that there are also pharmacies and long-term services and support and other clinics that are embracing this movement and going for, or have received, designation.

Expanding upon the current successes, however, it was acknowledged that the work is ongoing so that smaller healthcare clinicians operating outside of larger health systems in other parts of the state have more awareness of age-friendly initiatives: "We have a lot of smaller hospitals and clinics across the state that may not even be aware of the age-friendly initiative. . . . How do we expand this out to beyond those large health systems?"

In the public sector, participants spoke to the potential value of the One Utah Health Collaborative. This governor-initiated, community-owned nonprofit public/private collaborative is focused on improving beneficial health outcomes for Utahns through increased access to behavioral health care, expanded scope of an Intensive Outpatient Clinic, and proactive health and wellness supports (Napier-Pearce 2022). Despite having heard about this group, little was known about any of the group's efforts related to age-friendly ecosystems. One participant stated, "That's a group that's trying to be innovative. There's a lot of powerful leaders up there. I don't know if there is that voice on that collaborative to speak to this, maybe there already is." Another participant suggested that this group could be "a facilitator to the collaboration between multiple healthcare systems and community agencies to really provide those sorts of services and support for our community members."

Beyond this Collaborative, other important stakeholders included Utah's Department of Health and Human Services (DHHS) and statewide collaborations with different county programs.

> I was in a meeting on Monday, and we were talking about our strategic planning. I've learned a lot about all of the people in the different programs for the health department that work together to try and promote what we do. There are a lot of people involved, but there's still gaps. There's still a lot [who] don't get the information.

Falling under the purview of Utah's DHHS, Area Agencies on Aging and nonprofit agencies that have healthy community designations were described as important stakeholders:

> As a nonprofit, we have a healthy community designation where we get local government—mayors, city councils—to work on policy-system, environmental change strategies and

> connect with all these sectors; there's a lot of potential stakeholders within that healthy community space.

With the alignment of shared goals, these entities were considered to be well situated to collaborate and most quickly advance change and age-friendly initiatives.

University Leadership, Faculty, and Students.

Related to discussions of healthcare stakeholders, participants identified the education of clinicians and healthcare leaders to be an important ingredient to the promotion of an age-friendly ecosystem. Training the next generation of healthcare clinicians, however, would require curricular revisions to update course content:

> There are organizations that help develop curriculum to educate our medical professionals. . . . It needs to start in some cases being able to train and prepare our healthcare professionals to provide primary care. . . . When was the last time [that curriculum] was touched? I know there's multiple chronic conditions out there that haven't been modified in decades, and that's unfortunate because you get healthcare providers that then come out with very little experience or knowledge.

Beyond educating the next generation of clinicians, participants described the role of schools in "educating the citizenry" and questioned whether education systems are addressing issues of aging and ageism within general education and diversity courses. Indeed, research continues to suggest that ageism remains a more acceptable and invisible "ism" compared to other sources of stereotyping, prejudice, and discrimination (Applewhite 2019; Nelson 2005). Without shifting these pervasive perspectives, age-friendly initiatives will be stunted and undervalued. The inclusion of age-related issues within the curriculum across disciplines was one suggestion for involving "university students as stakeholders because they're the up-and-coming burgeoning planners of cities and planners of services and managers of grocery stores." Participants suggested developing a general education course on aging to be taken by all students: "What an important course. Everyone in any of the majors could be a stakeholder—health care, architecture, law, business—they all should really be aware of issues surrounding aging." As seen at the University of Massachusetts Boston, which began endorsing Age-Friendly University principles in 2017, some gerontology courses have been designated as qualified to meet students' general education requirement for diversity coursework (Silverstein et al. 2019). General education coursework on aging could be interdisciplinary and discipline specific (Obhi et al. 2019) or designed as an interprofessional or service-learning course (Howell et al. 2021; Mulvaney et al. 2020).

Education of the general population was envisioned to include stakeholders across all education levels, including elementary, middle, and high school, as well as all institutions of higher education across the state (perhaps to be convened by the Utah System of Higher Education). Doing so would benefit from the diverse resources available in other institutes of education. In addition, as described by one participant, "I grew up in a society [where] we are always taught to respect our older adults. . . . We have to bring that back, that respect; and plant that seed when children are in elementary school, middle school, and high school."

Participants encouraged conceptualizing stakeholders beyond students to include the entire campus community—administrators, deans, faculty, and staff. While creating age-friendly campuses may not be a typical priority for institutions of higher education, there was discussion of the role of campuses serving as "anchor institutions" in their communities:

> Increasingly we're being asked to serve a role that some people call "anchor institution" so that we have a larger mission to the communities in which we exist. And so, there is increasing recognition that we have resources that can do additional things beyond the educational and research missions that we have.

Also included in discussions of stakeholders were retired faculty members who were identified as stakeholders not to be ignored in age-friendly efforts. At the University of Utah, there is a Professors Emeriti Club who "have been incredibly supportive [of age-friendly initiatives] and, frankly, they've been senior vice presidents of faculty affairs and they've been senior vice presidents of health sciences. So, they have a really good, clear focus on how to move forward." The two-way utility of volunteer retired educators was described by participants who felt that volunteer work would provide older volunteers a sense of purpose:

> Educators have to educate, so my best volunteers are [retired] educators because they're passionate about it. So, I think that those people will have energy and passion and be able to help. They are key stakeholders and that also does a service to them because.. .you've got to have a purpose in your life if you want to keep on living. And so, we need each other. Let's use that group.

Finally, alumni and local philanthropists were identified as potential donors, and thus important stakeholders, to support the facilitation of age-friendly campus initiatives. As recognized by prior age-friendly planning efforts, program sustainability over the long term is tied to ongoing financial investments (Russell et al. 2022). Key to facilitating donor investment was education and promotion of age-friendly initiatives given the general perception that "aging isn't seen as one of those top priorities that we need to focus on." Nevertheless, one participant agreed that "there are certainly people who want to help. And so, giving them ideas on how they can help and opening their eyes to these concerns with aging—we can maybe help facilitate that. It's not a bad idea."

Businesses, Religious Groups, and the General Public of All Ages

Conceptualized as a public setting outside one's home (a "first place") and work or school (a "second place"), a "third place"offers a setting for informal gathering and connection to acquaintances (i.e., those to whom older adults may have "weak ties" as compared to the stronger ties to close family or friends) (Oldenburg 1999). Third places can include community facilities, local businesses, or green spaces and have been found to contribute to older adults' social engagement and, as a result, to higher subjective well-being and self-reported health (Sugiyama et al. 2023). Related, workshop participants described the persons in these spaces as stakeholders—retailers, banks, libraries, grocery stores, and pharmacies, including those that deliver, especially for "people who have a tougher time getting out." Businesses were described by workshop participants as having the capacity to support older adults' transitions into retirement and identification of activities in later life:

> We all recognize if we don't stay active, retirement means the next step is the six feet under. You've got to keep going; you've got to keep active; you've got to have a reason to be and people who lose that purpose deteriorate, I think. And so, businesses can help in people's transition. . . . What can we do to help facilitate your next step—whatever that may be?

The benefit of becoming a stakeholder for older adults was further described as coming with a financial reward for industries willing to work toward meeting the needs of a diverse aging population:

> People [aged] 50-plus contribute $7 trillion in annual spending. And so, another stakeholder that we need to think about is that the industry benefits from an age-diverse population if they know how to connect with them; who's providing those services and [who will benefit from] an age-diverse population?

Religious and cultural groups were also recognized as sources of informal support and social engagement for older adults, and thus valuable stakeholders: "The socialization aspect, or the opportunities to interact to gain social support; if you can't access services online, you need a neighbor to help you; and then opportunities for civic engagement. I think churches provide that opportunity." While religious communities were identified as useful at the neighborhood level for group members, if someone is not a member it can cause a barrier to inclusion:

> Church groups. . .do a really good job. . .making sure that all populations, especially and including the disabled and aging individuals. . .in the neighborhood. . .are aware of what's going on. I think we probably don't put as much into recognizing church groups as we should, and I think they do a great job at taking care of their populations. So maybe that's a focus we can work on a little bit more. Maybe that would be something that would be beneficial, working with church groups.

Opportunities for social and civic engagement have long been recognized as supportive of older adults' health and well-being (Herzog et al. 2002; Serrat et al. 2020), even if the mechanisms of action remain unclear (Jenkinson et al. 2013). Similarly, perceived disconnection is reduced among older adults who participate in social or community events (Cao et al. 2020). Thus, as neighborhoods, health systems, and campuses work toward age-friendly initiatives, important stakeholders for consideration include those who offer "weak" or informal ties to older adults and can support older adults' engagement and participation in social actions.

Older Adults

Perhaps evidence of unconscious ageism (Weiss and Lang 2012), older adults were explicitly mentioned only briefly and only by a few workshop participants as stakeholders in the age-friendly ecosystem. Though only a brief mention of older adults was made, all the above categories of stakeholders include older adults, as well as individuals who will be older in the future. One participant stated, "I might add to the list of stakeholders older adults, and citizens themselves. The neighbors, neighborhood people, the public, however you want to call us." Though many did not specifically cite older adults, participants put forth notions that the general populace should be regarded as stakeholders: "People in our communities. If we are all demanding these changes and demanding this age-friendly ecosystem, it will speak volumes." Nevertheless, prior research on developing age-friendly efforts has described the necessity of involving older adults, though older adults' participation could range from passive to active engagement (Rémillard-Boilard et al. 2017). Thus, depending on the goals for different age-friendly initiatives, older adults' participation might range from receiving information about initiatives to consultation, involvement, and collaboration in developing and designing initiatives, to empowerment to lead initiatives (Rémillard-Boilard et al. 2017). Depending on which engagement level is pursued, effective engagement will require age-friendly information across a variety of digital and non-digital platforms, as well as time and financial resources to sustain engagement over the long term (Rémillard-Boilard et al. 2017). In addition, as older adults who are healthier or have more social resources may be more able to participate or lead efforts, age-friendly initiatives should aim to include voices from marginalized and vulnerable groups, ensuring representation of older adults with diverse backgrounds and varying abilities (Buffel and Phillipson 2016; Menec and Brown 2022).

Conclusion

As communities, health systems, and campuses increasingly adopt upstream approaches to supporting older adults, age-friendly initiatives have blossomed. Consequently, there is a good deal of evidence on the actions that can best support older adults to age well and thrive. However, there remains a need for diverse stakeholders to commit the time, energy, and resources to the age-friendly ecosystem rather than competing initiatives. Recruitment of new stakeholders to age-friendly efforts are needed to encourage society-wide shifts in perceptions of aging. And while one workshop participant stated, "If you think about it, who isn't a stakeholder?" there could be an argument made that if everyone is seen as a stakeholder, then perhaps no one is. Thus, age-friendly champions and leaders are needed throughout the ecosystem as representatives for advancing age-friendly initiatives, collaborating across sectors, and involving older adults in the process. By including these diverse community voices in the planning and decision-making processes—for neighborhoods, health systems, and campuses—there are increased opportunities to support the development of age-friendly spaces for all.

References

Applewhite, A. 2019. *This Chair Rocks: A Manifesto Against Ageism*. Celadon Books.

Avey, P.C., and M.C. Desch. 2014. What Do Policymakers Want From Us? Results of a Survey of Current and Former Senior National Security Decision Makers. *International Studies Quarterly* 58 (2): 227–246.

Brown, J., K. Homer, and D. Isaacs. 2009. The World Café. In *The Change Handbook: The Definitive Resource on Today's Best Methods for Engaging Whole Systems*, ed. P. Holman, T. Devane, and S. Cady, 179–194. San Francisco, CA: Berrett-Koehler Publishers, Inc.

Buffel, T., and C. Phillipson. 2016. Can Global Cities Be 'Age-Friendly Cities'? Urban Development and Ageing Populations. *Cities* 55: 94–100. https://doi.org/10.1016/j.cities.2016.03.016.

Burow, P.B., K. McConnell, and J. Farrell. 2019. Social Scientific Research on the American West: Current Debates, Novel Methods, and New Directions. *Environmental Research Letters* 14 (12): 125012. https://doi.org/10.1088/1748-9326/ab4030.

Cao, Q., H.I. Dabelko-Schoeny, K.M. White, and M.S. Choi. 2020. Age-Friendly Communities and Perceived Disconnectedness: The Role of Built Environment and Social Engagement. *Journal of Aging and Health* 32 (9): 937–948. https://doi.org/10.1177/0898264319865421.

Farrell, T.W., W.W. Hung, K.T. Unroe, T.R. Brown, C.D. Furman, J. Jih, R. Karani, P. Mulhausen, A.M. Nápoles, J.O. Nnodim, G. Upchurch, C.F. Whittaker, A. Kim, N.E. Lundebjerg, and R.L. Rhodes. 2022. Exploring the Intersection of Structural Racism and Ageism in Healthcare. *Journal of the American Geriatrics Society* 70 (12): 3366–3377. https://doi.org/10.1111/jgs.18105.

Fouché, C., and G. Light. 2011. An Invitation to Dialogue: 'The World Café' in Social Work. *Qualitative Social Work* 10 (1): 28–48. https://doi.org/10.1177/1473325010376016.

Fulmer, T., P. Patel, N. Levy, K. Mate, A. Berman, L. Pelton, J. Beard, A. Kalache, and J. Auerbach. 2020. Moving Toward a Global Age-Friendly Ecosystem. *Journal of the American Geriatrics Society* 68 (9): 1936–1940. https://doi.org/10.1111/jgs.16675.

Hamel, L., A. Kirzinger, C. Muñana, and M. Brodie. 2020. *COVID-19 Vaccine Monitor: December 2020*. Retrieved from https://www.kff.org/coronavirus-covid-19/report/kff-covid-19-vaccine-monitor-december-2020/

Herzog, A.R., M.B. Ofstedal, and L.M. Wheeler. 2002. Social Engagement and Its Relationship to Health. *Clinics in Geriatric Medicine* 18 (3): 593–609.

Howell, B.M., L.C. Redmond, and S. Wanner. 2021. 'I Learned That I Am Loved': Older Adults and Undergraduate Students Mutually Benefit From an Interprofessional Service-Learning Health Promotion Program. *Gerontology & Geriatrics Education* 42 (2): 252–267.

Jackson-Elmoore, C. 2005. Informing State Policymakers: Opportunities for Social Workers. *Social Work* 50 (3): 251–261.

Jenkinson, C.E., A.P. Dickens, K. Jones, J. Thompson-Coon, R.S. Taylor, M. Rogers, C.L. Bambra, I. Lang, and S.H. Richards. 2013. Is Volunteering a Public Health Intervention? A Systematic Review and Meta-Analysis of the Health and Survival of Volunteers. *BMC Public Health* 13 (1): 1–10.

Menec, V., and C. Brown. 2022. Facilitators and Barriers to Becoming Age-Friendly: A Review. *Journal of Aging and Social Policy* 34 (2): 175–197. https://doi.org/10.1080/08959420.2018.1528116.

Mulvaney, E.A., R. Jantea, P. Leslie, P. Toto, M. Allias, C. Grant, V. Hornyak, J. Klinger, R. Nelson, S. Skledar, K. Covaleski, and R.M. Wright. 2020. Improving the Interprofessional

Practice, Knowledge, and Skills of Health Professions Students Through an Interactive Course in Gerontology. *Advances in Social Work* 20 (2): 184–203.

Napier-Pearce, J. 2022. Gov. Cox holds signing event for the One Utah Health Collaborative. *State of Utah, Office of the Governor*. Retrieved from https://governor.utah.gov/2022/09/06/gov-cox-holds-signing-event-for-the-one-utah-health-collaborative/

Neal, M.B., A.K. DeLaTorre, and P.C. Carder. 2014. Age-Friendly Portland: A University-City-Community Partnership. *Journal of Aging and Social Policy* 26 (1–2): 88–101. https://doi.org/10.1080/08959420.2014.854651.

———. 2015. From Planning to Implementation for an Age-Friendly Portland. *Public Policy & Aging Report* 25: 23–27. https://doi.org/10.1093/ppar/pru054.

Nelson, T.D. 2005. Ageism: Prejudice Against Our Feared Future Self. *Journal of Social Issues* 61 (2): 207–221.

Obhi, H.K., J.A. Margrett, Y. Su, S.L. Francis, Y.-A. Lee, D.A. Schmidt-Crawford, and W.D. Franke. 2019. Gerontological Education: Course and Experiential Differences Across Academic Colleges. *Gerontology & Geriatrics Education* 40 (4): 449–467.

Office of the Governor. 2019. *ReiMAgine Aging: Planning Together to Create an Age-Friendly Future for Massachusetts*. Retrieved from https://www.mass.gov/doc/age-friendly-ma-draft-action-plan-january-2019/download

Oldenburg, R. 1999. *The Great Good Place: Cafes, Coffee Shops, Bookstores, Bars, Hair Salons, and Other Hangouts at the Heart of a Community*. Da Capo Press.

Rémillard-Boilard, S., T. Buffel, and C. Phillipson. 2017. Involving Older Residents in Age-Friendly Developments: From Information to Coproduction Mechanisms. *Journal of Housing for the Elderly* 31 (2): 146–159. https://doi.org/10.1080/02763893.2017.1309932.

Russell, E., M.W. Skinner, and K. Fowler. 2022. Emergent Challenges and Opportunities to Sustaining Age-Friendly Initiatives: Qualitative Findings From a Canadian Age-Friendly Funding Program. *Journal of Aging and Social Policy* 34 (2): 198–217. https://doi.org/10.1080/08959420.2019.1636595.

Serrat, R., T. Scharf, F. Villar, and C. Gómez. 2020. Fifty-Five Years of Research into Older People's Civic Participation: Recent Trends, Future Directions. *The Gerontologist* 60 (1): e38–e51. https://doi.org/10.1093/geront/gnz021.

Silverstein, N.M., M. Hendricksen, L.M. Bowen, A.J. Fonte Weaver, and S.K. Whitbourne. 2019. Developing an Age-Friendly University (AFU) Audit: A Pilot Study. *Gerontology & Geriatrics Education* 40 (2): 203–220. https://doi.org/10.1080/02701960.2019.1572006.

Sugiyama, M., H.-W. Chau, T. Abe, Y. Kato, E. Jamei, P. Veeroja, K. Mori, and T. Sugiyama. 2023. Third Places for Older Adults' Social Engagement: A Scoping Review and Research Agenda. *The Gerontologist* e-pub:1–13. https://doi.org/10.1093/geront/gnac180.

Weiss, D., and F.R. Lang. 2012. They' Are Old But 'I' Feel Younger: Age-group Dissociation as a Self-protective Strategy in Old Age. *Psychology and Aging* 27 (1): 153–163. https://doi.org/10.1037/a0024887.

Chapter 7
Age-Friendly Futures: Equity by Design

Valerie Chang Greer and Linda S. Edelman

Chapters in this book have explored dimensions of age-friendly ecosystems (Fulmer and Huang), focusing on the contexts of neighborhoods (Hong), universities (Montepare, Farah et al.), and health (Felsted and D'Antonio). Insights are gained through specific consideration of the Intermountain West where a symposium and World Café was convened to consider the design of physical and social means to advance equity in aging well (Canham and Farrell). Chapter authors demonstrate how the goals and objectives of age-friendly places are knit into the physical realms of place and are supported by social programming and networks of relationships. Additionally, chapter authors highlight the active role that the invisible injuries of ageism play in shaping experiences of aging. While there are clear and important distinctions between what supports aging well in the realms of neighborhoods, campuses, and health environments, we recognize that places are not static entities, but in a constant state of flux and that there are inherent differences between histories, cultures, and contexts tied to place, which makes strategies to promoting age-friendliness site specific. Given the diversity of places, people, and contexts, and the heterogeneity of older adult populations, we celebrate the grassroots nature of the age-friendly movement which has historically built on processes of engaging people at local levels to generate knowledge and action. We recognize, as we face a landscape of widening disparities in health, that inequities in aging are not "natural" phenomena but the result of social, economic, and political constructions. An ecosystem model of age-friendliness thus provides a critical framework for

V. C. Greer (✉)
College of Architecture and Planning, School of Architecture, Healthy Aging and Resilient Places Lab, The University of Utah, Salt Lake City, UT, USA
e-mail: valerie.greer@utah.edu

L. S. Edelman
College of Nursing, Hartford Center of Geriatric Nursing Excellence, Utah Geriatric Education Consortium (UGEC), Utah Rural Opioid Consortium Collaborative Care Model (UROHC-CCM), The University of Utah, Salt Lake City, UT, USA

V. Chang Greer, L. S. Edelman (eds.), *Age-Friendly Ecosystems*, SpringerBriefs in Public Health, https://doi.org/10.1007/978-3-031-68361-9_7

holistically addressing questions of health that are not tied to single locations, but rather are embedded in the many places we live across our lifespan. Moreover, the work to create age-friendly ecosystems opens an important platform to examine health disparities across a range of contexts and advance equity and age inclusivity through the realm of design.

This chapter examines the role of design and participatory engagement processes in advancing equity in aging. It is significant that the age-friendly movement recasts older adults as active participants in coproducing visions for age-friendly places and moves beyond traditional, top-down approaches that view older adults as "customers expecting services" (van Hoof et al. 2021). The focus on co-production and social engagement is critical to future directions that address disparities in aging and broaden a discourse on equity to impact all ages. We turn attention to intersectional frameworks of research justice and participation (Bailey et al. 2019; Gilmore-Bykovskyi 2022) as well as design processes that leverage more diverse, nuanced, and inclusive perspectives on aging toward creative processes (Handler 2018). We also consider the integration of age inclusivity with broader diversity, equity, and inclusivity efforts in the contexts of neighborhoods, campuses, and health systems. Finally, we consider the question of measuring impact among historically marginalized and underrepresented populations. Having examined why an age-friendly ecosystem is important, and what the impact of age-friendliness looks like within the context of neighborhood, campus, and health environments, this chapter brings forward ideas on how future work can address the widening disparities in aging and promote a "more experimental, participative, and empowering engagement with people's possible relationships" to spaces where they age (Handler 2018). We begin by recognizing a common theme to recast aging and broaden conceptualizations of stakeholders, then we revisit socially engaged processes that aim to promote age-friendly places, and finally, we consider how to define and measure progress across a variety of settings.

Recasting Aging

In preceding chapters, authors addressed how age-friendliness can result in positive outcomes across the lifespan. Age-Friendly Ecosystems, as proposed by Fulmer and Huang (this volume), include five sectors: public, health systems, cities and communities, employers, and universities. We (Greer and Edelman) propose in Chap. 2 that when Age-Friendly Ecosystems embrace diversity and inclusion, they will become more resilient across all sectors. Conversely, ageist stereotypes and attitudes result in society viewing the contributions of older adults negatively, limiting the positive and meaningful contributions older adults may make to communities. It is significant to note this theme runs throughout place-types within neighborhoods, campuses, and health systems.

Aging, even as a natural concept, is often couched as a negative asset to individuals and societies. Ageism which includes stereotyping or discrimination based on age is well entrenched in modern culture. In the United States, we revere "the now"—i.e., modern buildings, new technology, and youth culture—and within this framework, aging has become a problem to fix, whether through programs or biomedical advances. Further, this contemporary and cultural view of aging contributes to implicit bias and discrimination that impacts almost every facet of the lives of older adults. This is particularly true when ageism intersects with other "isms" such as gender, race, and sexuality.

Older adults themselves fall prey to ageism, engaging in lifestyle choices—such as moving into 55+ communities, disengaging from popular culture, and embracing anti-aging products—that perpetuate stereotypes. Therefore, in the future, it is important that we change how individuals view their own subjective aging, or how they make sense of their own aging process (Westerhof et al. 2014). By reframing their views of subjective aging to be more positive, older adults can improve functional health, well-being, and even live longer (Levy 2009). In fact, one longitudinal study that followed adults 50 years of age and older for over two decades found that those with positive self-perceptions of aging lived 7.5 years longer than those with more negative self-perceptions (Levy et al. 2002a, b).

The intersection of aging and other areas of discrimination such as gender, race, and disability impacts how societies, communities, and individuals experience aging. Older women historically are more likely to experience poverty and live in nursing homes than older men (Older Women in Poverty 2018; Mudrazija et al. 2015). People of color, because of lifelong disparities in access to care, have more chronic illnesses at younger ages and have shorter life expectancy (Quiñones et al. 2019). These intersectionalities were exacerbated by the COVID-19 pandemic. Older adults of color, or those with more functional limitations, were disproportionately at risk of dying from COVID. Healthcare supplies and workforce shortages at a time when older adults needed more intense care to treat COVID-19 infection led hospitals to consider how resources were allocated. Concerns that categories such as advanced age and predicted life-years saved were going to exclude older adults categorically from treatment options resulted in the American Geriatrics Society publishing a position statement that included avoiding age alone as a means for denying care (Farrell et al. 2020). The statement also addressed the need to consider how biases related to race, ethnicity, and sociodemographic factors amplified disparities in health that resulted in increased comorbidities (Farrell et al. 2020).

How can aging be recast to promote healthy aging? We propose that the Reframing Aging initiative launched by the Leaders of Aging Organizations in 2014 to "improve the public understanding of older people's needs and contributions to society" (D'Antonio 2020) be used to change the language we use about aging to be positive and, thus, build "a groundswell for change—from local efforts to national leaders—to tell a more balanced story of aging" (https://www.reframingaging.org/) that can impact all Age-Friendly Ecosystems sectors—public health, health systems, cities and communities, employers, and universities.

The Reframing Aging Initiative aims to effectively advocate for older adults by using language that is inclusive, focuses on solutions, and avoids negative language that generalizes physical decline or incapacity as normal aging. By reframing aging through a positive lens, a new shared language can be developed to talk about aging that avoids negative assumptions and sets older adults apart (D'Antonio 2020).

Instead, reframing can "help people see aging as a continuous process and to recognize that older age, like any other time in life, involves both opportunities and challenges" (Finding the Frame 2017) Reframing Aging best practices include (1) using inclusive language that is free of age bias; (2) highlighting the diversity in the older population by avoiding broad categorizations; (3) talking positively about changing age demographics and avoiding catastrophic terms; (4) emphasizing collective responsibility and social context; (5) talking about aging as dynamic process with benefits to society; (6) defining ageism to increase realistic perceptions of aging; (7) including concrete, systems-level solutions; and (8) incorporating the concepts of justice (all people are treated equally) and ingenuity (people are resourceful and can find creative solutions to aging challenges) (Communication Best Practices 2022).

For many years, the aging population has been couched in negative terms—the aging tsunami, the greying of America—that represent older adults as consumers of resources, not producers, and aging as a problem to be solved. By focusing primarily on the challenges that an aging population has on programs such as Social Security and Medicare, we ignore the fact that many older adults remain active engaged participants in their communities and families until late in life. When we reframe the narrative of aging to address the contributions of older adults and provide systems-level solutions, we avoid fatalism and encourage people, including older adults, to embrace programs and policies that support the aging population (Communication Best Practices 2022). More importantly, movements such as the Reframing Aging Initiative and the Age-Friendly University Global Network encourage and support older adults to remain actively engaged in their communities.

Social Engagement and Diversity in Aging

One of the most significant characteristics of the age-friendly movement is its inductive, "ground-up" approach to identifying social and environmental factors that support aging well. Age-friendliness means different things in different geographical locations and settings, and while there are common categories such as transportation, housing, and social participation, the contexts of unique cultures, resources, and infrastructure render paths toward age-friendliness as being distinct based on place. The context of what supports age-friendliness in Salt Lake City, Utah, is entirely different from what might be found in Singapore, which is radically different again from that in Stockholm. While age-friendliness represents a global movement on one level, we understand its core building blocks begin in places and contexts that are inherently different from each other. Factors which support age-friendliness are rooted in the milieu of place and are not necessarily transferable. Cross-cultural dialogue and knowledge exchange are promoted through platforms such as WHO's AFCC database. Industry-based sectors, such as the American Academy for Gerontology in Higher Education (AGHE) in higher education and the Institute for Healthcare Improvement (IHI) in healthcare delivery, play a critical role in promoting awareness, resources, and learning across professional networks in different geographical locations. Yet age-friendliness inherently resists a universal, "one-size-fits-all" set of strategies, which may be simultaneously the most brilliant and the most bedeviling part of the movement. As such, community engagement processes are foundational to the ability to connect to particular places, cultures, and contexts in age-friendly work.

Significant to the grassroots or "ground-up" nature of age-friendly ecosystems is the work to build and encourage inclusive language that honors diversity, avoids "us versus them," and includes older adults as creators of solutions to address aging. This reframing occurs by design and intentionality. When inequalities are addressed, older adults, regardless of socioeconomic status, have access to resources and technology; they can access information and communicate with younger generations, thus empowering them to be active voices in their communities. When the narrative includes older adults of all gender identities, races and ethnicities, and abilities, communities become aware of the unique strengths and positive contributions of older adults collectively. This reframing in turn decreases ageism and increases community engagement.

Looking ahead, we submit that it is necessary to radically reposition community engagement at the heart of age-friendly work in order to address issues associated with inequities in aging. Given the great polarities that are experienced financially, socially, and health-wise among *all* adults, it is imperative to widen the lens and the approaches to centering community engagement processes in order to not just represent the well resourced but to especially account for the challenges faced by historically marginalized and underrepresented people. Socially engaged practices and processes are unique to locations; however, the infrastructure of widening the lens can lead to radically different perspectives; this needs to be prioritized in order to recognize the diversity of experiences and to be meaningful to those most in need.

We hope readers of this book will leave with the question of "age-friendly for whom?" The stark reality is that disparities in aging are compounding and may be outpacing the important work of the age-friendly movement. We believe the next generation of age-friendly work must be rooted in a deep commitment to address inequities in aging, which begins with community engagement processes designed to create visibility and action around inequities in aging.

In tandem with the needs of a dynamic and diverse aging population, there is a critical opportunity for the age-friendly movement to be further integrated with work and policies that address larger economic, environmental, and health issues posed by rapid urbanization, homelessness, climate change, and mental health crises. Inequities in aging are inextricably entangled with a broader spectrum of global issues, which are manifested on regional levels in unique ways. Understanding design challenges to creating age-friendly ecosystems requires cross-disciplinary work as the myriad obstacles we face today are, in many ways, unprecedented. In order for age-friendly work to be truly impactful and responsive to contemporary conditions, there is a need to lock arms with those working in other fields to address the wicked problems of our time. To quote Ashton Applewhite in "This Chair Rocks" (p. 12)—"When we make the world a better place to grow old in, we make it a better place in which to be from somewhere else, to have a disability or be queer or non-white or non-rich." Here, social engagement is essential to coproducing knowledge and action.

Fostering Intergenerational Relationships

A radical repositioning of community engagement opens doors for a more inclusive focus on identity and inclusion among older adults, as well as a broader set of issues to address with healthy aging. It is time to double down on creating truly inclusive engagement processes in order to generate new knowledge and networks of action that are essential to creating and sustaining age-friendly ecosystems. One way of addressing healthy aging in the context of age-friendly ecosystems is through intergenerational experiences and relationships within the community and through higher education.

In today's culture, close intergenerational relationships outside the family are rare, even though more generations are working together (Mcpherson et al. 2001; Lahey 2008). This lack of intergenerational connectedness is in part to the lack of age-integrated neighborhoods (Winkler and Klaas 2012). While most communities include members of all ages, the interconnectedness between generations is often lacking without intentional efforts to bridge them. In other words, age-friendly communities must be more than built environments and concepts such as universal design that foster healthy aging. They must also create intergenerational opportunities that bring generations together in meaningful ways. To do this, engaging the voices of all residents in community initiatives, and intentionally designing programs that support intergenerational relationships, is important. The intergenerational connections that result can benefit older adults (improved health and quality of life, reduced social isolation and loneliness) and children and youth (improved social skills and school performance and better choices) (https://www.gu.org/app/uploads/2018/05/SignatureReport-Eisner-INeedYou-Background-Paper.pdf).

It is also imperative that intergenerational relationships are fostered in higher education to benefit both younger and older students. As the population ages, the need for healthcare clinicians committed to caring for older adults is going to continue to increase. Past experiences with older adults can influence students' attitudes about aging and interest in working with older adults in their future careers. Medical students who have more interactions with older adults also have more positive attitudes, making them more likely to consider geriatrics as a career (Voogt et al. 2008). Nursing students are more likely to have positive attitudes toward older adults if they have past rewarding experiences with older adults or if they are provided with service learning or simulation activities that include older adults in their curriculum (Magan et al. 2023). The Age-Friendly University initiative promotes intergenerational learning which benefits younger students, including reducing negative stereotypes and creating more positive attitudes (Gautam et al. 2023). The benefits of intergenerational learning for older students include feeling more connected to younger generations and improved self-esteem.

Measuring Progress

The WHO's Decade of Healthy Ageing 2020–2030 focuses on global efforts to support individual countries to develop healthy aging strategies through the collection of global data, the development of standardized measures of aging, and collaboration and data sharing to develop healthcare systems that address the needs of older adults across settings. Healthy relationships with place are instrumental to healthy aging. The World Health Organization defines healthy aging as "the process of developing and maintaining the functional ability that enables well-being in older age" (https://www.who.int/news-room/questions-and-answers/item/healthy-ageing-and-functional-ability). This definition centers the role of place, as "functional ability," and encompasses a multitude of mechanisms that allow people to meet basic needs, to be mobile, to learn and grow, to nurture and maintain relationships, and to contribute to society. The WHO definition of healthy aging also invites a need to build shared language and understanding which recognizes intersectionality as a critical component that informs how people "function" within many types of spaces. Yet another dimension of the WHO definition of healthy aging is that it compels us to broaden our thinking about the benefits of regular physical activity and decreased sedentary time. A 2022 Annual Review by Dogra and others identified five health outcomes (physical function, cognitive function, mental health, social health, and sleep) that can be targeted by increasing physical activity levels. While most efforts to increase physical activity have focused on behavioral change, Dogra et al. (2022) propose creating communities through age-friendly policy and design that are universally accessible encourage intergenerational social engagement, and facilitate physical activity can improve these health outcomes. In addition, technology can be used to enhance mobility, from individual mobile devices to smart cities and homes that use data to promote physical activity.

Chapters of this book speak to the shared need for data that measures and tracks the impact of age-friendly neighborhoods, campuses, and health systems on health and well-being. While individual organizations that contribute to aging have systems of measurement, it is a separate challenge to track collective efforts which come together to measure the impact of age-friendly places and initiatives. For instance, if one wanted to understand the resources that promote nutrition and healthy food choices for older adults in any given area, they might look at the work of Meals on Wheels, which tracks the number of meals provided, number of older adults served, etc.; however, understanding the broader impact of resources on health, nutrition, and aging well within any given community requires also understanding transportation options, food costs/subsidies, resources provided through senior centers and health clinics, etc. Much of the work of creating age-friendly places aims to work upstream of health complications, i.e., preventing chronic diseases such as diabetes and obesity through healthy food choices for older adults, which present other challenges including organizational continuity and access to longitudinal data. Increasingly, there are efforts to measure and track the impact of preventative measures including the physical and social environment, but the funding and knowledge required to sponsor these efforts is scarce. Political will must come together with public awareness in order to support the mechanisms for funding this important work. Additionally, there is a need for mixed methods as a means of assessment; data that uses smart technology and other means of generating quantitative data is a frontier that needs further exploring.

There are three paradoxical conditions within contemporary discourse about design for aging which should be addressed within the discussion about measuring impact. The concepts of "universal design," "inclusive design," or "design for all" are inherently utopian (Bianchin and Heylighen 2017); there is a tipping point where widening the definition of these terms to be inclusive for some becomes restrictive or prohibitive for others. This paradox of inclusion reflects the utopian nature of aspiring for universality and compels us to question what it means to design for the widest possible audience. Additionally, there is a paradox of participation. Older adults, who tend to spend the most amount of time in places like their neighborhoods, are often among the least engaged and underrepresented in the decision-making process (Buffel et al. 2018). The traditional focus on research and problem-solving through designing for older adults often belies the ability of older adults to be agents in the production of place (Handler 2018). New approaches to age-friendly design might move beyond a "baseline of objective needs" and into reconsidering the roles of older people themselves in relationship with the places they live. Finally, there is the paradox of engagement, which is that age-friendliness tends to be on the agendas of policy-led discussions, yet has remained limited in the discourse on aging and urbanism within design discourse (Handler 2018; Noordzij et al. 2019). This points to the need for urban practitioners, including architects, designers, and artists, to engage with the policymaking community (Buffel et al. 2018). Recasting the role of community developers, health and social care professionals, designers, researchers, and policymakers in relationship to the variety of participatory methods needed to draw out a diversity of information from the lived experiences of older adults (Buffel et al. 2018; Gilmore-Bykovskyi et al. 2022; Handler 2018). The paradoxes of inclusion, participation, and engagement are distinct from each other and should be addressed in defining measurement tools.

Future work will be well supported by recognizing and addressing current challenges to measuring impact. Quantitative and qualitative data is needed to assess the range of ways that age-friendly places shape health and well-being. Documenting and sharing methods are essential in order to promote learning across sectors, as well as across cultures and contexts.

Conclusion

The global and US populations are aging. While society often views this demographic shift negatively, this chapter focuses on the many initiatives that are addressing aging positively. Historically, ageism has been the invisible "ism"—the "only -ism in which we act against our future selves" (Nelson 2005)—resulting in interpersonal, self-directed, and institutional inequities against older adults. In this chapter, we bring attention to positive initiatives, such as Reframing Aging, that are combating ageism and propose work to be done to make, as Terry Fulmer proposes in Chap. 1, age-friendly ecosystems the norm. Initiatives such as the Gerontological Society of America's Reframing Aging Initiative are bringing attention to ageism through the use of positive narratives to change public perceptions of aging. By including health equity and equality in the narrative, we are able to bring awareness to how the intersectionality of aging with other vulnerabilities negatively impacts aging across the lifespan and helps age-friendly places—whether communities, health systems, or universities—support healthy aging for all people. Fostering intergenerational relationships within families, communities, and workplaces can increase the visibility of older adults, improving their sense of connectedness and self-worth, and help build a tapestry of connections that positively impact younger generations as well. Building integrated and inclusive age-friendly ecosystems can strengthen individuals, families, and communities.

References

Bailey, J., V. Steeves, J. Burkell, L.R. Shade, R. Ruparelia, and P. Regan. 2019. Getting at Equality: Research Methods Informed by the Lessons of Intersectionality. *International Journal of Qualitative Methods* 18: 1609406919846753.

Bianchin, M., and A. Heylighen. 2017. Fair by Design. Addressing the Paradox of Inclusive Design Approaches. *The Design Journal* 20 (sup1): S3162–S3170.

Buffel, T., S. Handler, and C. Phillipson. 2018. *Age-Friendly Cities and Communities*. Bristol: Policy Press.

Communication Best Practices. 2022. *Reframing Aging Initiative Guide to Telling a more Complete Story of Aging*. https://www.reframingaging.org/Portals/GSA-RA/images/RAI%20Communication%20Best%20Practices%20Guide%20220328.pdf?ver=yoPyMu-AfQLqH9ZuzKqjNw%3D%3D

D'Antonio, P. 2020. Reframing Aging: A Generation's Work. *Innovation in Aging* 4 (Suppl 1): 723. https://doi.org/10.1093/geroni/igaa057.2559.

Dogra, Shilpa, David W. Dunstan, Takemi Sugiyama, Afroditi Stathi, Paul A. Gardiner, and Neville Owen. 2022. Active Aging and Public Health: Evidence, Implications, and Opportunities. *Annual Review of Public Health* 43 (1): 439–459.

Farrell, Timothy W., Lauren E. Ferrante, Teneille Brown, Leslie Francis, Eric Widera, Ramona Rhodes, Tony Rosen et al. 2020. AGS Position Statement: Resource Allocation Strategies and Age-related Considerations in the COVID-19 Era and Beyond. *Journal of the American Geriatrics Society* 68 (6):1136–1142.

Finding the Frame: An Empirical Approach to Reframing Aging and Ageism. 2017, February. A FrameWorks Research Report.

Gautam, R., S. Sritan, M. Khumrungsee, and K.D. Melillo. 2023. Promoting Age-Friendly University by Engaging Older Adults in Intergenerational Learning at Institutions of Higher Education: PRISMA-Guided Scoping Review. *Journal of Intergenerational Relationships*: 1. https://doi.org/10.1080/15350770.2023.2251467.

Gilmore-Bykovskyi, A., R. Croff, C.M. Glover, J.D. Jackson, J. Resendez, A. Perez, and J.J. Manly. 2022. Traversing the Aging Research and Health Equity Divide: Toward Intersectional Frameworks of Research Justice and Participation. *The Gerontologist* 62 (5): 711–720.

Handler, S. 2018. Alternative Age-Friendly Initiatives: Redefining Age-Friendly Design. In *Age-Friendly Cities and Communities*, 211–230. Policy Press.

Lahey, J.N. 2008. Age, Women, and Hiring: An Experimental Study. *Journal of Human Resources* 43 (1): 30–56. https://doi.org/10.3368/jhr.43.1.30.

Levy, B. 2009. Stereotype Embodiment: A Psychosocial Approach to Aging. *Current Directions in Psychological Science* 18 (6): 332–336. https://doi.org/10.1111/j.1467-8721.2009.01662.x.

Levy, B.R., M.D. Slade, and S.V. Kasl. 2002a. Longitudinal Benefit of Positive Self-Perceptions of Aging on Functional Health. *Journals of Gerontology, Series B: Psychological Sciences and Social Sciences* 57: P409–P417.

Levy, B.R., M.D. Slade, S.R. Kunkel, and S.V. Kasl. 2002b. Longevity Increased by Positive Self-Perceptions of Aging. *Journal of Personality and Social Psychology* 83: 261–270.

Magan, K.C., S. Ricci, and E. Hathaway. 2023. Factors Influencing Baccalaureate Nursing Students' Attitudes Toward Older Adults: An Integrative Review. *Journal of Professional Nursing* 47: 1–8. https://doi.org/10.1016/j.profnurs.2023.03.012.

Mcpherson, M., L. Smith-Lovin, and J.M. Cook. 2001. Birds of a Feather: Homophily in Social Networks. *Annual Review of Sociology* 27: 415–444.

Mudrazija, S., M.B. Thomeer, and J.L. Angel. 2015. Gender Differences in Institutional Long-Term Care Transitions. *Womens Health Issues* 25 (5): 441–449. https://doi.org/10.1016/j.whi.2015.04.010.

Nelson, T.D. 2005. Ageism: Prejudice Against Our Feared Future Self. *Journal of Social Issues* 61: 207–221. https://doi.org/10.1111/j.1540-4560.2005.00402.x.

Noordzij, J.M., M.A. Beenackers, A.V.D. Roux, and F.J. van Lenthe. 2019. Age-Friendly Cities: Challenges for Future Research. *Bulletin of the World Health Organization* 97 (6): 436.

Older Women in Poverty. 2018. Justice in Aging. https://www.justiceinaging.org/wp-content/uploads/2018/12/Older-Women-and-Poverty.pdf

Quiñones, A.R., A. Botoseneanu, S. Markwardt, C.L. Nagel, J.T. Newsom, D.A. Dorr, and H.G. Allore. 2019. Racial/Ethnic Differences in Multimorbidity Development and Chronic Disease Accumulation for Middle-Aged Adults. *PLoS One* 14 (6): e0218462. https://doi.org/10.1371/journal.pone.0218462.

van Hoof, J., H.R. Marston, J.K. Kazak, and T. Buffel. 2021. Ten Questions Concerning Age-Friendly Cities and Communities and the Built Environment. *Building and Environment* 199: 107922.

Voogt, S.J., M. Mickus, O. Santiago, and S.E. Herman. 2008. Attitudes, Experiences, and Interest in Geriatrics of First-Year Allopathic and Osteopathic Medical Students. *Journal of the American Geriatrics Society* 56 (2): 339–344. https://doi.org/10.1111/j.1532-5415.2007.01541.x.

Westerhof, G. J., Miche, M., Brothers, A. F., Barrett, A. E., Diehl, M., Montepare, J. M., Wahl, H. W., & Wurm, S. 2014. The influence of subjective aging on health and longevity: a meta-analysis of longitudinal data. *Psychology and Aging, 29* (4): 793–802. https://doi.org/10.1037/a0038016

Winkler, R., and R. Klaas. 2012. Residential Segregation by Age in the United States. *Journal of Maps* 8 (4): 374–378. https://doi.org/10.1080/17445647.2012.739099.

Index

V. Chang Greer, L. S. Edelman (eds.), *Age-Friendly Ecosystems*, SpringerBriefs in Public Health, https://doi.org/10.1007/978-3-031-68361-9

GPSR Compliance
The European Union's (EU) General Product Safety Regulation (GPSR) is a set of rules that requires consumer products to be safe and our obligations to ensure this.

If you have any concerns about our products, you can contact us on

ProductSafety@springernature.com

In case Publisher is established outside the EU, the EU authorized representative is:

Springer Nature Customer Service Center GmbH
Europaplatz 3
69115 Heidelberg, Germany

www.ingramcontent.com/pod-product-compliance
Lightning Source LLC
Chambersburg PA
CBHW071716101125
35216CB00019B/901
9783031683602